T0150753

THRIVE IN YOUR
HEALING BUSINESS

Advance Praise

"A fantastic, beautiful, and much-needed book. Heather writes with passion and clarity coupled with deep and broad experience as a healer, and her work will make yours—whether on yourself or with your clients—not only easier but much more meaningful. A heads up to all my coaching colleagues: you'll be getting this book for the holidays this year!"

–**Liza Baker**, Health Coach and
Founder of the (Sorta) Secret Sisterhood

"Heather's book is inspiring, informative and 100% what every healer who is feeling burned out needs. She generously shares her own story, the lessons she has learned along the way and her phenomenal program in this book. Her teaching is easy to understand and just as easy to assimilate and integrate into your journey. With honesty, vulnerability and a charming sense of humor Heather teaches you everything you need to have the healing practice you have always dreamed of having. I highly recommend this book for anyone in the healing arts."

–**Rob Meyer-Kukan**, Founder of the
Healthy Musician Institute

"*Thrive in Your Healing Business* left me feeling inspired and motivated. I really enjoyed Heather's recommendations of practices, skills, and tools for personal and professional development. The chapter on money was particularly helpful in reframing pricing and how it is part of the message we as teachers and healers send. This book was everything I was hoping for and much more!"

—**Leila Bordo**, Healing Movement Specialist

"Heather shares her own journey with love and care. This book is a joy to read! It helped me realize that I wasn't alone with my own struggles in my business. Throughout the book, Heather offers practical insight and tools for self-care. By using the tools that she teaches in this book I feel that I can be of greater service in the world."

—**Jill C Brown**, Advanced Life Coaching

"This book is a valuable resource to help any healer thrive in their role. Whether just starting or a seasoned practitioner, the tools in this book are practical, accessible, and actionable. The CLARA and FORWARD methods can be applied to any life situation to help us move through resistance and trust our decisions. *Thrive in Your Healing Business* will move you from a burnt-out rescuer to an empowered server to those who need you!"

—**Chris Ce**, Author of *Get the F*** On with Your Life: Healing After a Toxic Relationship*

"Heather Glidden inspires me as a healer to take better care of me in order to improve my life and practice. *Thrive in Your Healing Business* is a step by step guide to success and happiness for healers, something we all need. Well worth the read!"

—**Kristi Brower**, Author of *Relationships for Spiritual People*

"All healers need to read this! I felt as though Heather was speaking directly to me in this book—what she writes resonates so much with what I experience in running a healing business. I will read it again and again."

–Anne Thomasson, Owner of
Gyrotonic St Louis Central

THRIVE
IN YOUR
HEALING
BUSINESS

Do the Work You Love
Without Sacrificing Yourself

HEATHER GLIDDEN

NEW YORK

LONDON • NASHVILLE • MELBOURNE • VANCOUVER

THRIVE IN YOUR HEALING BUSINESS
Do the Work You Love Without Sacrificing Yourself

© 2020 HEATHER GLIDDEN

Published in New York, New York, by Morgan James Publishing in partnership with Difference Press. Morgan James is a trademark of Morgan James, LLC.
www.MorganJamesPublishing.com

ISBN 978-1-64279-515-8 paperback
ISBN 978-1-64279-516-5 eBook
ISBN 978-1-64279-540-0 Audio
Library of Congress Control Number: 2019902398

Interior Design by:
Bonnie Bushman
The Whole Caboodle Graphic Design

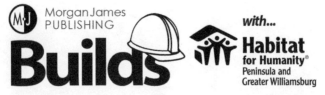

In an effort to support local communities, raise awareness and funds, Morgan James Publishing donates a percentage of all book sales for the life of each book to Habitat for Humanity Peninsula and Greater Williamsburg.

Get involved today! Visit
www.MorganJamesBuilds.com

This book is dedicated to my husband Matt.
Thank you for your unwavering support
through this entire journey.

TABLE OF CONTENTS

FOREWORD

In today's world the healing profession is thriving. Despite this, many healing professionals are finding themselves burnt out from their meaningful work. I'm excited to share that *Thrive in Your Healing Businesses* closes this gap by offering you an engaging and comprehensive approach to self-care.

As a motivation scientist and sustainable-behavior-change coach, I have spent decades studying what allows people to create lasting self-care behaviors. I've found that the reasons why we are told we "should" do something like take better care of ourselves tend to fail because they give us a one-size-fits-all approaches and meanings for self-care that emphasize *future* goals pertaining to our medical health and/ or weight.

Yet, emerging research suggest that adopting self-care behaviors that we can sustain necessitates cultivating a meaning for self-care that deeply connects with who we each are and what we value, *today* rather than tomorrow. But how can professionals change their embedded frame of reference and approach self-care in this new way?

Thrive in Your Healing Businesses offers just this guidance. Through stories and easy-to-implement practices, you will receive Heather's wise teachings about how to leverage your resistance, uncover you own personal meaning for self-care, and also learn concrete "how to's" of making your own self-care a daily priority and strategy.

By integrating insights from spiritual traditions with specific strategies, Heather gives us a one-of-a-kind guide to help professionals in the healing arts create a meaningful and effective approach to their own self-care; one that will permit them to do their very best work while also cultivating time for themselves and their families.

Compassion fatigue and burnout have become epidemic. In this insightful and inspiring book, Heather Glidden gifts us the core beliefs and essential practices that healers of all kinds can use to prevent or address burnout so they can thrive instead of just survive.

—**Michelle Segar**, Bestselling Author of
*No Sweat: How the Simple Science of Motivation
Can Bring You a Lifetime of Fitness*

CHAPTER 1

ON THE OUTSIDE, EVERYTHING LOOKS GREAT

"I feel like this is my life's work, but I just don't know if I can keep doing it anymore," Sidney tearfully admitted to me.

Sidney was a nurse who was in the process of transitioning into full-time work as a life coach. She had an infectious smile and a determined ability to find the good in any situation. She had come to her work as a coach after her husband had suffered a serious injury. Every day for years, she would envision him recovering, even though the doctors said it couldn't happen. When he finally did recover, in a way that seemed almost miraculous, she felt in her gut that her visualization had made that happen.

But life didn't return to normal after his recovery. She realized that she had envisioned him healthy, but she hadn't envisioned happiness. "I was expecting the healing to give him back," she said, "but it didn't fix things—my visualization had been for healing; not for happiness."

She began visualizing happiness, allowing it to unfold without expectation for how that would look. Over time, she began to see the results. She felt happier, her husband felt happier, and they enjoyed their life with their two sons.

After going through this, she realized that she wanted to share the healing she'd experienced with other people.

"It took a lot of years for me to realize why I had suffered for so, so long—now I can look back and see why. It happened so I can connect with other people. I want them to know that we have the ability to create the life we desire through our thoughts and actions," she told me.

She had taken a life coach training and was ready to build a coaching business to help other people heal and create the lives they truly desire.

I'd been working with her on building her coaching business for a couple of months, and things were going great! She was getting invitations to speak and even finding reservoirs of wisdom to share that she'd never expected she had. She'd been asked to share her message of positivity and empowerment with a local massage therapist's clientele. She'd been invited to speak at a symposium with hundreds of her ideal clients in the audience.

At her boss's retirement party just two weeks earlier, she'd spontaneously given a speech about her boss's impact on her life and the power of people in leadership positions to shape an organization. Everyone was crying by the end of her speech, and management had invited her to a conversation about how she could offer coaching to affect the direction of the organization.

On the outside, it looked like everything was going great. She was building the business she wanted and sharing the message she so wanted and needed to share.

But on the inside, she felt like she was about to have a nervous breakdown. Between working with her coaching clients, juggling her job as a nurse, and trying to be a good mom and wife, she was getting pulled too thin. She was losing her temper with her kids, losing the connection she'd worked so hard to rebuild with her husband, and she had no quality time for herself.

"I keep Googling for retreats or vacations, but I just want to go by myself! I feel so guilty saying that, but I can't be the caretaker for everyone right now. When my kids and husband are with me, I feel like I still have to be in the caretaker role," she said.

She admitted that she felt like a fraud, sharing this message of hope and empowerment with the world when her own life felt so out of control. She noticed that she started to resent it when people asked her for help.

"Normally, I just want to give and caring comes naturally for me. But now I feel like I can't even care," she said. "What if I'm not cut out to be a healer?"

She came to me for help to get her business and her healing work in control so she could enjoy her life again. Even though she was afraid that she might not be cut out to be a healer, she still desperately hoped that she could make it work. But between all the pressures of her work, her husband, and her kids, she knew she was going to need support.

My heart went out to her, as it does for every healer who finds themselves in this situation. It is a dark, sad, lonely place to be.

But the good news is that I have learned, both through my own experience and through working with my clients, how to balance a healthy life with a healthy healing business!

I've actually come to believe that this is a critical phase that every healer must go through at some point on their healing path. In learning how to balance your role as a healer with the rest of your life, you must do a lot of your own powerful healing work. This allows you to be a more effective healer.

I taught Sidney what I'm going to teach you. It allowed her to create the balance that she was craving so she could have quality time for herself and her family while still doing the work she loved. Getting her life in balance didn't require a lot of time or a vacation to Bali. It was actually a lot simpler than she thought it would be, and it changed everything in how she related to her business.

I wrote this book as a love letter to every healer who finds themselves in that dark, lonely place. If that is you, please know that you are not alone! You can do the healing work that calls your soul and also live a healthy and well-balanced life. This book will show you what I've learned about how to do that.

CHAPTER 2

IT'S NOT ABOUT
THE BUSINESS MODEL

M y first nudge toward this work came very early in my
career in the form of a movement client. Dr. Robert
was a well-respected holistic doctor in my community. As a
new teacher offering an obscure movement method called
the Gyrotonic system, I couldn't believe he wanted to work
with me!

I had not yet stepped into the title of healer for myself,
but it was something I very much aspired to. Working with
such a well-known and well-respected healer felt like being a
young actress and getting a gig with George Clooney.

Every Friday afternoon, he would come in for his lesson
after his last patient of the day, and I would set him up for
a series of movements called "Hamstring Series." In the
Hamstring Series, the client's legs are supported using a

weighted pulley system, so they feel almost weightless. It's a relaxing way to start a session, and after a full day of being on his feet treating clients, he was so ready for it.

He would begin doing the movements and with each repetition he would get slower… and slower… and slower. His breath would get deeper. Some weeks he actually fell asleep, and some weeks he merely got close. Either way, the message was clear: He was exhausted.

As we worked together more and I got to know him better, I began to see the high toll that his healing work took on him, both physically as well as emotionally. I saw how it had strained his relationship with his wife and seemed to have taken over his whole life. He was always quite honest about this.

One day he told me, "You're a very talented young healer, but if you are going to make a living of this, it's not enough to just do the work. You'll have to figure out how to take care of yourself too."

I was equal parts elated and sobered. On the one hand, I had just received genuine validation of my healer credentials from an unassailable source. I'd arrived! On the other hand, I realized how right he was.

As a movement teacher, I often worked with people in their fifties, sixties, or seventies who had pain or other chronic injuries. What I frequently noticed was that the ailments these people experienced had roots in some event or habit from their early adulthood. I could clearly see that if they had addressed this issue in their twenties, thirties, or forties it would have been much easier, faster, and less costly to correct.

I rapidly extrapolated this insight out to my whole life and decided I would not become a burned-out healer. I would learn the secrets to healer self-care early so I could avoid that particular pitfall entirely.

What I think the Universe heard when I made that bold statement was, "Hey Universe, I want to learn everything there is to learn about healer burnout, and I want to learn it on a really accelerated timetable. Please fast-track me for some tough-love self-growth lessons!"

And let me tell you this: Always be careful what you ask for. Because you will get it.

Another benefit of working with Dr. Robert turned out to be that he was a great referral source. Before I knew what had happened, I had a full-to-overflowing clientele of people, most of whom had significant injuries or health concerns. As I helped them get better, more and more came.

I left the studio where I had been renting equipment and opened my own studio. Within the same year, I grew to a staff of five, expanded the new studio, and attended an 800-hour massage program to give me more tools to help my clients.

Within two years of opening my studio, I was completely burned out. I was teaching six days per week, six to ten hours per day. When I went home, I was managing emails and coordinating with my staff. I often stayed at my computer until midnight. I hardly saw my husband. I hardly saw my friends.

And the worst part was that the work I had found delightful and engaging only a couple of years earlier just felt flat to me. I would struggle to stay awake through lessons and count the hours till I could go home each night.

I knew I couldn't keep going like that, so I started searching for solutions. I noticed that I would get a boost of energy and inspiration after attending a training, so I started taking more trainings. Of course, trainings cost money, so when I was home, I still needed to work just as much in order to be able to afford the next training.

When I look back on this time now, it looks like an addiction to me—always saving up for the next hit and hoping it would get me through until I could afford the one after that.

After a couple of years using that strategy, I could feel it getting less effective, so I started looking for the next thing that would keep me going. I decided to partner with another woman to run the studio, hoping that if I had less studio work to do then I would feel more refreshed in my teaching work.

In order to create the partnership, we merged our two studios, creating one much larger studio. It turns out, and perhaps this shouldn't have been a surprise to me, that having a much larger studio is much more work. So of course, you can see that I wasn't out of hot water yet. Moreover, there were new conflicts involved in the new partnership.

I started having panic attacks. I spent my entire thirty-fifth birthday curled in my bed hyperventilating. I remember another time when I was hiding in a closet at my studio shaking uncontrollably and telling myself, "You have a client in five minutes. I don't care how you do it, but you have to pull yourself together *now*."

Somehow, I always did pull myself together for my clients. To the world, I looked like I had a successful business and like everything was under control. But inside, I knew it was an act—one that I couldn't sustain. The longer I wore that mask, the more it felt like my soul was dying.

"Obviously, I just need to teach less. If I teach less, then my life will feel more spacious, and I'll be happier and feel better about everything," I thought. It sounded very logical.

So I hired a business coach who helped me revamp my business model so I could make more money while teaching fewer hours. I finally had free time!

But a strange and totally surprising thing happened once I had free time. I had no idea what to do with it! I had no idea who I was when I wasn't working. I felt more anxious than ever before.

I ended my partnership and built a new studio. I was determined that I would finally get it right this time. I was going to build the studio around the concept of joy, and it would finally give me what I had wanted from my work for so long.

Can you guess what happened? Of course, the studio didn't give me joy. Weird catastrophes started happening. The husband of one of my instructors suddenly decided he wanted a divorce. She moved out of town as a result, and we were left short-staffed. Our landlord suddenly decided that he didn't want us to put a sign on the front of the building. Despite having a highly visible location on Main Street, we couldn't get any traction on awareness-building campaigns. It was the hardest I'd worked on a studio in my life, and I was getting fewer results than I'd ever had.

Every day I asked myself, "What's wrong with this studio? The whole plan for this studio was to feel more joy, and the dang thing is just making me more miserable than ever!"

It was in my grief after one of my instructors whom I dearly loved had told me that she just couldn't stay anymore and she was leaving to work at another studio that it finally clicked.

Before this point, I had learned all the pieces I needed in order to make my work sustainable for myself— the marketing, the business model, the scheduling, the boundaries, the delegating—but I was missing the one key piece that I needed to bring it all together and make it sustainable.

The studio wasn't going to bring me joy, and I had to stop expecting it to do that.

Changing my schedule wasn't going to make my life feel spacious.

Going to trainings wasn't going to make my teaching inspired—not in a lasting way.

All of those things had to come from inside of me. Learning how to create the internal state that I desired—to be the joy, the spaciousness, the inspiration—was the final step. I had to learn how to tap into that place inside of me before I could sustainably create balance in my life.

I tell you all of this because I want you to understand that my own journey to balance my healing work with my life has been long and circuitous. I'm not writing this book as a passive observer. I can only share this knowledge from a place of having lived it. I feel like I learned every lesson in this book the hard way, often multiple times, to get to the point where I could confidently know that I can create this balance for myself and also lead others in creating it for themselves.

I don't know if this will make sense yet, but if you are craving true balance in your healing business and life, then you will have to get this sooner or later. You can make all the changes on the outside that you want—and you may need to do things like changing your rates or your working hours—but none of that will ever make a true and lasting difference until you learn how to actually create that internal state for yourself first.

If it was as easy as just changing your hours, you would have done it already.

Once you learn how to create the internal state that you desire, everything changes. Once I learned how to be joyful and spacious and inspired—that I could actively choose those states regardless of outside circumstances—then I was able to start seeing all the ways that I had actually chosen to create the opposite situations for myself. And of course, then I was also able to start making new choices.

What changed for me? On the outside, it probably looked like very little changed. Unlike all of my other attempts to solve the problem, this one didn't come with big external changes at first. I think many people in my life probably didn't even realize anything different had happened.

But on the inside, I finally felt free in a way that I hadn't felt for years. I took more delight in my work and in my time off. I felt calmer, and I discovered that I was more powerful than I ever, *ever* suspected was possible. My panic attacks ended, and a whole host of other minor health issues cleared up.

I had always expected that the solution to balancing my healing business with my life would be something very clever: just the right business model or marketing plan or schedule. But one day, I realized that I hadn't changed any of those things (although some were in the process of evolving), yet I had fallen into balance.

Over the years, I've met with so many other healers and colleagues who have struggled to balance their business with their lives. Once I made this discovery, I knew I needed to share it.

In working with my clients, I've found that it's not necessary to go through nearly so many difficult lessons as I went through in order to get your business under control and enjoy quality time for yourself and with your family (thank goodness!). That's why I've written this book. It is my very dear wish that it will help you to find the balance and sanity that you are craving!

CHAPTER 3

LEARNING TO WALK

Paul scowled in concentration as he slowly moved his legs through an exaggerated walking pattern—carefully coordinating his timing so one leg reached forward as the other one pushed back. When I finally told him he could rest, he collapsed with an exclamation of, "Why the heck is something that looks so easy so dang hard?!"

Paul came to me to help him resolve long-standing low back pain. His doctor had told him he needed to work on strengthening his core, and he had an image of doing some kind of fancy sit-ups. When I told him we were going to practice walking instead, he gave me a look like I was a little crazy. Obviously, he could already walk—how did I think he'd gotten himself into my studio?

I explained to him that it's the activities we do every day, often completely unconsciously, that often lead to chronic pain. I took a short video of him walking and showed him how his low back arched every time he took a step. In a healthy gait pattern, the glutes should fire to propel you through space, but in his walking pattern, all of the stress was going into his low back. Once I showed him his pattern, he realized how learning to walk correctly could have a huge impact on how his back felt.

So the answer to curing his back pain was very simple: He just needed to learn how to walk correctly!

However, as Paul soon learned, simple is not the same as easy. In the beginning, every time he tried to do the movement of taking a step, he went straight into his low back. He had to allow me to passively guide his leg before it was even possible for him to feel the new pattern. Then he had to do the movement very slowly, with one leg at a time until he could feel the difference between the correct movement and his old pattern. Then he needed to practice the movement with both legs at the same time, still supported so he could do the movement slowly. Finally, after all of that (which took months), he was able to notice that his gait pattern was naturally changing, even when he wasn't at the studio.

I told you in the last chapter that the techniques needed to balance your healing business with your life are quite simple, and they are. But, like Paul learning to walk again, simple doesn't necessarily mean easy.

What you must do in order to successfully create balance in your life is to create a new habit, and that takes practice, dedication, and often, guidance. What made it so difficult for Paul to learn how to walk correctly? Well, he had a lot of practice with his old pattern! By my guess, he probably had thirty-forty years of practice at walking by arching his low back. He was a complete expert at it, and I was asking him to learn, and apply habitually, an entirely new pattern.

If you've found that your business and life are out of balance, then that is a pattern too. The longer it's been like that, the more habitual it is. In fact, once you start to become aware of the underlying forces that have brought you to this place, you will probably realize that they have roots in habits that started long before you even started your business. This is why it takes a process (similar to the process I used to help Paul learn to walk correctly) to create new and healthy habits for how you relate to your business.

A New Path

You must start by setting the pattern you wish to follow. For example, you might want to set new patterns of spaciousness, joy, and balance. We must begin by helping you to cultivate these qualities in your own life, as it exists right now.

This will probably feel very backward to you. I find with most of my clients (and I had this belief myself for a long time) that they think they need to create more space in their lives and then they will feel more spacious. I have watched friends and colleagues go for years and years saying, "This is just a really crazy time but, as soon as things calm down, then I will…"

I am going to tell you a big truth right now: If you are waiting for things to calm down before you allow yourself to feel calm and sane, they will never slow down. You can choose to believe me or not, but I promise you that if you try it, you will see what I mean. The world just doesn't work like that. The next drama will always be waiting around the corner. If you don't believe me, then keep waiting for a bit longer, but pay attention. Notice how one wave always follows the next.

This is because you are in the habit of living your life this way. The outside world is responding to your internal state.

It is very difficult to see this while you are in it. I was actually never able to see this in my life until one of my mentors made a video of me and showed me. Just like with Paul and the walking, I wasn't able to see it until I had the perspective of looking from the outside.

Once I saw it, I could never go back to how I'd been. It took a lot of practice and a lot of support, but I was able to create a new pattern for myself. I was able to learn how to be spacious, how to be joyful rather than waiting for the world to give me those experiences. Gradually, the world around me began to reflect those choices.

Make It a Habit

Paul's back pain didn't go away because he practiced in my studio. It went away because he took what he learned in my studio and made it a habit in his everyday life. It will be the same for you and your business.

The first step is to practice your new state of being in an isolated and supported way, but sooner or later, you will need to learn how to create it in any situation. This is how you truly and sustainably change your life. This is how you put your practice into action!

You must be able to create a state of spaciousness even when the bills are due or your kids are screaming or you just got an email from a client that left you super triggered.

This is where the real work starts. The more you incorporate this work into all areas of your life and the more you make it your habitual state of being, the more lasting the change will be. This doesn't happen overnight, but you will start to see the changes with each effort that you make.

The big key here is taking new actions. You cannot keep doing things the way you've been doing them and expect different results. As you move into a new state of being, you are going to realize that certain things don't work for you anymore. You might realize you need to change your hours. You might realize you need to raise your rates. You might discover you need to hold new boundaries. You might realize you need to fire some clients or have some other difficult conversations.

All of this is going to make you feel very uncomfortable.

The In-Between

Paul felt very uncomfortable when I was making him learn to walk again. To start with, he felt ridiculously embarrassed that, as a grown man, he needed to learn how to walk. And then he had to concentrate so hard to do what I was asking of him. And then he had to go through that awful stage when his old gait didn't feel good any more, but the new one didn't feel right yet either.

This is a critical stage! I call it the In-Between. It's kind of like the Upside Down in the show *Stranger Things*: Everything kind of looks the same, but it's not quite right, and it all feels a little creepy. It would have been so easy for Paul to say, "This is a load of hooey!" and quit. But he didn't. He stuck with it, and within a few weeks, he was on the other side. His new gait pattern felt more normal, and his back pain was already a memory of the past.

I can virtually guarantee that you will get to a point with this work where you will want to say, "This is a load of hooey!" and quit. It will come when things feel super uncomfortable and you are definitely out of your old habit, but the new one isn't set yet.

That is one of the many experiences I've selflessly had for you so that you needn't (unless you choose to) have the experience for yourself. Actually, looking back, I can see I've done this at least three times. In each case, things started to change very fast, and I got very freaked out. In my freak out, I started demanding that they *stop* and go back to how they used to be.

And you know what happened?

They stopped. They didn't really go back to how they used to be because you can never go back. You'll never again be the person you are right now. But I did end up spending a *lot* more time in the In-Between than I needed to. It was also harder to get moving again once I realized I really did want to get to the other side after all.

What I'm offering here has the potential to launch significant changes in your life. But it will test you, and you will have to choose whether you are truly ready make those changes.

The things that healers usually need to do to bring their lives into balance aren't complicated. For most of us, the answer is some combination of setting new boundaries around our hours or schedule, giving ourselves permission to delegate and let go of work that leaves us overextended, consistently making the space to release any energy we take on from our clients, setting our rates at a level that truly supports us, and acknowledging when it's time to move on to doing new work. None of this is rocket science. But there's a lot going on under the surface that determines whether we succeed at these goals.

Dr. Bruce Lipton, author of *The Biology of Belief*, states that up to ninety-five percent of our behavior is controlled at the subconscious level. Our subconscious beliefs are like a powerful undercurrent, constantly shaping our behavior. There are some shared subconscious beliefs that often send people into healing work, beliefs like, "I am only of value when I'm helping other people." And there are other beliefs that come in at the societal level like, "a healer shouldn't charge very much money for their services or else they will be considered greedy." In order to make true and lasting change, you must actually gain access to and address your own subconscious beliefs. If you've tried to make any of the changes I mentioned above and you haven't been successful, then this is generally the biggest missing piece I see that needs to be addressed.

Often people wait until their current situation is so painful that they can't possibly stay in it. That pain is the only thing strong enough to make them willing to go through the necessary discomfort of making real change. But it doesn't have to be like that. It's equally possible to move toward something. Maybe it's having more quality time for yourself. Maybe it's having better relationships with your family.

If you find yourself hesitating, ask yourself: What are you really afraid of? What are you ready to move toward? What are you willing to do in order to make that change?

Every overworked healer I've ever met has their version of what I call The Cabin. The Cabin is the place you fantasize about retreating to and becoming a hermit when it feels like you are caring for the whole world. It's not a cabin for everyone. For some, it's a beach or a mountain lake or a quiet grove of trees, or a meadow. For one notable exception, it was a Vegas casino. Regardless of how it looks, The Cabin is the place you fantasize about going to take care of yourself and where you don't have to take care of anyone else.

I drew pictures of my cabin. I vision-boarded my cabin. It was a little rustic place on a hillside, surrounded by trees. I imagined living there with some animals and having a little garden and never seeing people again. For years, I had this fantasy. Even though I knew at the same time that working with people is one of the top things that gives my life meaning and purpose, I still imagined that somehow I would never really be happy until I lived this complete hermit existence in a cabin.

I finally decided I would try it—but just as a trial. I wasn't ready to end my marriage and release all of my earthly belongings to live a hermit life in a cabin without at least giving it a trial run first. (Thank God!)

I spent many nights researching retreat centers and finally found one where I could stay at a little cabin in silence and solitude. It was a completely rustic cabin with no electricity and no heat beyond a wood-burning stove. It looked perfect!

I booked a week in the cabin, envisioning a peaceful, meditative retreat. I purposely chose a time when it would be cold outside so I could use the wood burning stove. I packed up my journals and my meditation cushions, kissed my somewhat bemused husband goodbye, and set off to explore my new life as a hermit.

The cabin was called The Hut, and it looked exactly the part I had envisioned. I lugged my suitcase up the hill to The Hut. (No cars allowed.) I put my journals on the desk. I set out my candles and a flashlight. I put my crystals on the windowsill as a little altar. It was going to be a perfect place to spend a week. I thought I would probably never want to leave.

I made it less than twenty-four hours.

It turns out that (and this really shouldn't have been a surprise to a girl who grew up backpacking in the Rocky Mountains) living in a rustic cabin when there is snow on the ground is *cold*. So, no problem, I had a wood burning stove, right? All I had to do was build a fire. I'd be toasty in no time.

Despite the doubts of my whole family, I actually had no trouble building a fire (they later gave all the credit to the wood—clearly it was good wood), but it took hours for the little cabin to heat up. And then I wanted to go to bed, but I was worried about the fire going out and the cabin getting freezing cold in the night again so rather than setting an alarm to get up in the middle of the night, I built the fire up really high. Now, the notebook in the cabin had specifically warned against doing this, but I thought, "It will probably be fine."

It was not fine. I woke up in the middle of the night in a sauna—dripping with sweat and choking on smoke. I ran around opening all the windows and begged the cabin to go back to being freezing.

Eventually, it cooled off, I got the fire going at a reasonable level, and the cabin got to be a comfortable temperature. That was about the time the sun rose, and it was time to get up. I was exhausted, my throat was rough from choking on smoke all night, and my romantic image of a peaceful life in a rustic cabin was completely in tatters.

I did actually make it one more night in the cabin, but full disclosure, this was only because I was informed that they had no other place to put me until the following day. The second night went better, but by that point I had already made a critical realization: I didn't need to be a hermit in a rustic cabin to have a happy life.

This was probably obvious to everyone else in my life, but I'm just wired in a way that I need to do things and prove them to myself before I believe them. So after that experience, I believed it.

But I'd had this image of the cabin for so long, and I still wanted to know: What was that all about?

What I came to realize was that the cabin wasn't a literal cabin. It was my mind and body's way of showing me what I really needed. I needed time in quiet, in solitude, in simplicity, in nature. My very soul was craving it, and the image it gave me so I could understand this was a rustic cabin.

The cabin wasn't mean to be a real and literal cabin; it was meant to be a pathway to a state that I could create for myself.

The subconscious mind works in this way: it offers images to help us know what we need but aren't really paying attention to.

Since then, I've noticed that my clients get images with similar messages: It's time to spend some time in nature, some time resting, some time alone.

If you have the resources, it can be great to actually take a beach vacation or get away to a mountain cabin (I recommend one with heat!), but what I've learned, both through my experiences and those of my clients, is that it's not actually necessary to go anywhere. You can take a retreat without ever leaving your house.

Close your eyes and picture the place that calls to you. Perhaps it's a meadow by a mountain lake, or perhaps it's a beach at sunset. Or maybe, like me, you imagine a cabin in the woods. Notice what the place looks like, how it feels. Who else is there (if anyone)? What does it smell like? What do you hear? Where do you feel like you most belong in this place? Notice as many details as you can about this place to make it as real for yourself as possible. Know that you can spend as much time as you need here, and you can return any time you want.

Reconnecting with Your Heart

Doing this work allows you to reconnect with and begin to heal your heart. The heart never stops talking, but when it says things we don't want to hear for long enough, we may cut the line. It takes attention and intention to re-open the connection. Doing something as simple as holding your hand on your heart, breathing, and wishing your heart well can start to re-establish the connection. Visiting your version of the cabin also allows the heart to heal.

This is especially important for healers because healing work is heart work. When you offer healing, you are working with heart energy. Healers generally follow their hearts into healing work, but at some point, it is easy to start feeling like we are responsible for doing the work rather than simply allowing healing to come through us. This is when we end up allowing ourselves to become overcommitted and burned-out. When we do this, we forget the fundamental nature of healing. Healing is something that comes through us, but we are the conduit not the do-er. The most important work in healing is the work of connecting to and following the heart.

The heart naturally knows how to replenish its own energy, but you must listen, and listening takes courage. All of the processes in this book are meant to help you reconnect with the messages of your heart, but you must decide if you have the courage to follow what it tells you.

I can promise that if you do, you will find yourself inspired and fulfilled in ways that currently seem beyond impossible.

I JUST WISH SOMEONE WOULD TAKE CARE OF ME!

"**I** work so stinkin' hard taking care of my clients all day, and then I go home, I cook a healthy meal for my husband, I help my son with his homework, and then I go to bed exhausted so I can get up the next morning and do it all again. I just wish someone would take care of me for a change!"

I was having lunch with a friend and colleague, and she was at her wit's end.

I could sympathize because I've been in the same place, and I've seen lots of other healers in that place as well. When we care for other people all the time, it can feel like we are all alone and no one takes care of us.

Here's the truth, though: Although we can always ask for help and support, we need to take care of ourselves first. If we aren't taking care of ourselves, how can we expect someone else to do it for us?

This is the shadow side of the healer archetype, and you must learn to recognize it if you want to build a sustainable and happy healing business.

Archetypes are roles that we play. For example, "mother" is an archetype. You may be a mother, but you aren't playing the role of "mother" all the time. When you go to work, you might stop actively playing the role of "mother" until you get home or you get a call from your kids. Alternatively, you might not have any children of your own, but there might be certain people for whom you play the role of "mother."

Archetypes are like the parts in a play. You can step into them and out of them. An archetype is not your job, although you may embody a certain archetype in order to do your work. If you picked up this book, then you are likely embodying the archetype of "healer" in your work.

Stepping into an archetypal role helps us to define our relationship to other people within the role. People will come to someone in a "healer" role for very different services than they would come to someone in a "warrior" role.

Every archetype has a light side—a side that gets expressed in a way that is beneficial to the person playing the role and those they serve—and a shadow side—a side that is detrimental to the person playing the role and those they serve.

The light side of the healer archetype expresses care and loving focus. It allows a spaciousness for life to unfold and natural order to be restored. There is a relaxed feeling to the light side of the healer archetype. A healer working in this space allows greater forces to work through them by working with the innate healing intelligence of the whole person in front of them.

The shadow side of the healer archetype tends to emerge when healers become overly attached to or involved in their work. This is when ego gets involved or the healer starts to over-identify with their work. Being in this aspect of the healer archetype feels draining. A few signs that you are working from this space are feelings of resentment, overwhelm, and burnout.

Remember that archetypes are roles we play. An archetype does not define who you are. If you find yourself expressing the shadow sides of the healer archetype, it doesn't mean that you are a bad person or a bad healer.

We all express our shadow sides. That is a part of life. What defines our experience is how effectively we can recognize when we are in that state, admit it to ourselves, and then work with it.

And that's the great news: You can shift yourself out of the shadow state! You can even learn a lot about yourself in the process.

But there's a challenge, and here we need to talk about being a martyr. "Martyr" is another archetype. Our society tends to celebrate martyrs, those who self-sacrifice in service of a cause. And like every archetype, "martyr" can have a light and a shadow side. There are times when a noble self-sacrifice comes from a place of pure service and may truly serve a greater cause. But because our society celebrates martyrs, it can be very easy to fall into playing this role from a place of ego or a desire to appear virtuous.

And if you go down this road, then it can be easy to start to feel like a part of your job as a healer is to be a martyr, as though you are not valued unless you are self-sacrificing in some way. I see this lead to healers who overwork themselves, who undercharge for their services, and whose other relationships suffer as a result. Over time, this leads to resentment and a victim mentality. And that's the challenge. Because as long as you think you are the victim, then you won't realize you have the power to change your own situation.

Let's look at this a little closer, and I'll explain why I think healers are especially prone to this challenge. If you can really master this, then you will not only be able to balance your own work and life; you will also become a much more effective healer, and you will find a richness in your relationships that you never knew was possible.

There is a cycle between victim and rescuer (and here I have to credit my own coach Heather Clark who first helped me see how this was at work in my own life). These are, again, archetypes. No one is born a victim or a rescuer; they simply play these roles.

As healers, we may cast ourselves in the "rescuer" role. In order for a "rescuer" to have purpose, they need a "victim" to help. So now we've cast our clients or patients in the role of "victim."

How is this problematic? Well, look back above at the description of the light side expression of a healer. Notice where the healing comes from in that situation. Is it the healer? No! The healer is creating the circumstances for healing to happen, but they aren't actually responsible for doing the healing.

So when a healer starts to get into the rescuer-victim dynamic, they are over-extending their own energy in a way that makes them look good ("look at me, I am the one who comes to the rescue"), but drains their energy and can actually block the natural healing that is available otherwise.

And what does this lead to? Well, an overextended healer is sooner or later going to become a victim who is now waiting to be rescued by someone else. It's a self-perpetuating cycle.

What if You Were to Serve?

So if we want to break this cycle of victim-rescuer and get out of the martyr mentality, we need to find a new approach. The new approach is to change the way you relate to your clients into one of service. Being in service enriches the healer and the client. It has an entirely different energy from the feeling of rescuing or self-sacrificing for someone else

Rachel Naomi Remen articulates this beautifully as the difference between serving and helping:

"Serving is different from helping. Helping is based on inequality; it is not a relationship between equals. When you help you use your own strength to help those of lesser strength. If I'm attentive to what's going on inside of me when I'm helping, I find that I'm always helping someone who's not as strong as I am, who is needier than I am. People feel this inequality. When we help we may inadvertently take away from people more than we could ever give them; we may diminish their self-esteem, their sense of self-worth, integrity and wholeness. When I help I am very aware of my own strength. But we don't serve with our strength, we serve with ourselves. We draw from all of our experiences. Our limitations serve, our wounds serve, even our darkness can serve. The wholeness in us serves the wholeness in others and the wholeness in life. The wholeness in you is the same as the wholeness in me. Service is a relationship between equals."

What I have seen, in my own life, and in the lives of my colleagues and clients, is that when we step into the intention of service with our clients, we step out of the victim energy and the shadow side of the healer archetype. And once we break that cycle, then we ourselves don't end up playing the victim role.

Try it on for yourself. Ask yourself, "How can I best help my clients?" It's easy to answer that question by saying, "I need to book sessions after hours. I need to charge less money. I need to offer them more of my energy."

And now try, "How can I best serve my clients?" When I ask that question, the first thing that I notice is how important it is for me to show up as the best version of myself! And I know I can't do that if I'm not living a balanced life, taking care of myself, and having good relationships outside of my healing business. It becomes so much easier, and so much more logical, to hold healthy boundaries and choose to care for myself.

Writing a New Story

If you've found yourself feeling like your healing business is running your life or out of control, then the first step is to recognize, with great love and compassion, that you've fallen into a martyr or victim story. Breaking out of this story takes really clear focus and intention. You need to know what story you are writing instead, but you also need to understand why you created this situation in the first place.

The victim mentality says, "I didn't create this situation. It just happened. Look at how much I'm suffering! If someone would take care of me, then I would be fine."

Notice how much that voice is asking for sympathy. It's asking for a rescuer. One of the benefits of being in this state is that people will feel bad for you. They will admire you for your "good work ethic." There is a perceived virtue to being in a martyr state.

There is also a cost. The cost is your health and wellbeing, your relationships, and, in my opinion, the true quality of your work because I think that one of the greatest services a healer can offer is empowerment, and a healer who is operating in a victim-rescuer mentality isn't self-empowered and so cannot offer empowerment.

A healer who is ready to take responsibility for having a balanced life says, "Wow, this is quite a mess I've created for myself. I feel like I'm about to have a breakdown. What changes can I start making to take better care of myself?"

Making this shift puts you in the driver's seat. No more waiting for someone to come to your rescue or wondering how much more you can take. Now you are in charge of your own life!

I'm not going to lie: It's scary making this shift. As long as you stay in victim mentality, then you can always blame someone else if things aren't going the way you want. Once you start taking responsibility, then the buck stops with you. If you don't like how things are going, then you know it's your responsibility to change them.

But living this way is also incredibly freeing and empowering. Once you break free of the victim-rescuer dynamic, you start to see so many more possibilities that you never noticed before.

Leave Me Alone!

One of my teachers, Atum O'Kane, says that sometimes you just need to tell your archetype, "I am a human being with a human life. You need to leave me alone right now."

I think this is a skill that all healers need to develop. It's easy to get overextended doing healing work. You have the golden trio of making money, making a difference in other people's lives, and looking good doing it because our society currently sees overwork as virtuous.

But you have a choice here, and what you need to get really honest with yourself about is what truly allows you to be most effective in doing your work in the world. How do you want to show up in your work and your life?

No one is going to rescue you. It's not your partner's job or your client's job. But you can rescue yourself! The first step is to shift how you look at the work you do and step into the light side of your healer archetype. Or even learn how and when to put the healer archetype down for a while.

If you're ready to have a new experience in your life and business, then it's time to write a new story for yourself. What do you want your new story to be?

CHAPTER 6
THE PRACTICE

N ow that you are ready to write a new story for yourself, let's get you the tools you need to do that. You are currently very practiced at the way you've been relating to your work and business. It's a strong habit. So you're going to need some practice at building a new habit.

The way to create more spaciousness in your life is to practice being spacious. The way to be more joyful in your work is to practice being joyful. The way to take a more empowered approach to your life is to practice making empowered choices.

All of this requires that you become aware of your old patterns so you will recognize them when they arise. I definitely recommend getting help for this part. We are so good at our patterns that they are always invisible to us at first. You'll need to find someone you can trust and who understands what you are doing to lovingly help you see when you're falling into your old patterns.

And then you will just have to practice, practice, practice with the new patterns that you want to create for yourself: patterns of empowered choices that lead to the life you truly want to be living.

You will backslide. You will have moments when you revert. You will put your foot in your mouth and screw up. You may be tempted to be harsh on yourself when you see these things happening, but in my world, all of this is great because it means you are trying new things. The goal here isn't to change your life and make it perfect overnight. I think we can both agree that isn't even possible, right? The goal here is to start making new choices and becoming aware of the moments when you slide back into your old habits.

You may have noticed that I've used the word "practice" already a lot in this chapter. That is because I want you to understand why this next tool is so important. The tool is to develop your own personal daily practice. In my opinion, this is the single most powerful tool you can use to create lasting change in your life.

Remember when I told you about how Paul had to learn to walk from scratch? That's you right now. You are learning how to walk from scratch. The first step is to give yourself a really safe, supported space to experiment. Don't start with trying to run!

Your daily practice is your safe, supported space to experiment. It's the gift that you give to yourself each day. It's putting on your own oxygen mask before you assist others.

Now, you may already have a daily practice, and if so, that's great! I'm going to make some suggestions for the practices I have found most effective in making this particular shift in your life and business. You may be able to incorporate them into the practice you already have, or you may choose to set aside a separate time to do them.

But I Don't Have Any Time!

I just wrote the word time above, and I thought I could almost hear you say, "But Heather, I'm here because I'm running ragged in my business! I don't have time to add a personal practice into my life!"

If that thought came up, then great! This is a great opportunity to do a little coaching right now. I want you to listen to that thought and see if you can feel the energy behind it. Is that coming from a place of empowerment? Is that something that a person who has chosen to be in control of their own life would say?

I'm hoping you can see that it is not.

If you feel like you don't have enough time for a personal practice, it is because you choose not to set aside the time for it. This is your first chance to make a new and empowered choice. If you want to experience more spaciousness in your life, this is an opportunity to choose to incorporate an experience of spaciousness every day.

You don't have to start with a long practice, although I recommend at least thirty minutes to truly start seeing benefits. Remember, this is about really making a commitment to yourself, and the time you spend needs to reflect that. Usually, I recommend putting your practice first thing in the morning as this helps to set your state for the rest of the day, although some of my clients prefer to do it before bed, and that works well for them. The most important thing is that you choose a consistent time and stick with it.

If you find yourself struggling to show up for your practice, I suggest this strategy that I've found super effective for helping myself and my clients. It's this: Do your practice first thing in the morning before even looking at your phone or email. If possible, do it before you even talk to anyone else. You are allowed to make coffee first if you are a coffee person—I get that question a lot! Just beware that you don't get distracted while the coffee brews.

A big part of what we are doing with your practice is helping you to get control of your own consciousness, and when you start your day with your phone or email, it's really easy to give that control away. By going to your practice before you do anything else, you are sending a message to the Universe and to yourself about what you prioritize, and that will have an effect through the entire rest of your day.

What Will Keep You Going?

This process requires discipline. There is no way around that. There will be times when you may want to hit the snooze button instead of getting up for your practice. There will be times when you have a to-do list a mile long, and it seems like you would be so much better off just skipping the practice. This is when you have to really use your discipline.

At this point, we need to look at what discipline means for you. When you hear the word discipline, what does it feel like for you? For me, discipline used to be associated with punishment or having to do things I really didn't want to do. I had to redefine discipline for myself. My new definition is the choice to commit to what is most important. I have a friend who defines discipline as, "a sacred appointment."

What definition can you use for discipline that will inspire you to maintain your practice? You'll always be more successful with your practice if you can reframe it in a way that makes you feel drawn toward it rather than pushed into it. What definition helps you feel drawn in to your practice?

A part of this process is knowing why you are making these changes. What matters most to you about balancing your life? And what matters about that?

I have a friend who recently ran a half-marathon. The race was at Disney World, and the reward for completing the race was a Millennium Falcon medal. That medal was his motivation. He knew he was going to finish the race to get that medal. But along the way in training for the race, he saw how much his health improved and also how he could be a role model for his kids and others in his life, and those realizations became his inspiration to make the actual training itself joyful.

What is your motivation (what gets you moving toward your goal) to make your work more sustainable?

And what inspiration (what gives your goal life and meaning) can you connect to along the way that will sustain you even when it's difficult?

What meaning does it have for you to make these changes in your life? What are the immediate benefits you will experience from staying committed to this process?

In her book, *No Sweat: How the Simple Science of Motivation*

Can Bring You a Lifetime of Fitness, Michelle Segar says, "When it comes to making a sustainable change in your behavior, understanding your *Meaning* is your starting place because it determines the tone of your relationship with [any behavior]. In practical terms, your Meaning… determines whether or not you will make time, day after day, to do it and ultimately whether you achieve your desired goal…"

My motivation for getting my business in balance was to spend more time with my family and to have more time for my own creativity. My daily inspiration is to show up as the best version of myself that I can every day, so I can do the best work possible for my clients. I do my practice to serve the work that I feel called to do in this world and to hopefully bring a little lightness into the lives of everyone I touch. In order to do that, I offer myself that light first.

When I approach it from that perspective, my practice always feels like a gift.

So, What Do I Do?

What goes into your daily practice?

This is something that you will refine over time, but I recommend starting with a two-part practice. Part one is a writing practice, and part two is a meditation practice.

I recommend starting with only the writing practice for the first week.

For your writing practice, you are going to do twenty minutes of stream-of-consciousness writing. Write down whatever is in your head. It might be lists of what you plan to do that day; it might be a tirade about something a client said to you the day before that has you really riled up; it might be really boring; it might not make any sense. Some days, my pages are full of sound effects and things that aren't even real words. Let it be whatever it is without a need to change it.

You may be tempted to slow down or try to make sense of what you are writing or make it sound good, but resist that temptation. As much as possible, just keep writing, and don't let yourself stop for the full twenty minutes.

This is where you unload everything that is in your head. It may seem pointless or silly, but really pay attention to your days during the first week that you practice this. Most people who undertake this practice notice a significant shift in how their days go within the first week of practice. Once you start seeing that shift, then you can use that inspiration to help propel you into adding the next piece of the practice: meditation.

Meditation can help you increase your focus and concentration, make clearer decisions, improve your creativity, and gain better access to your intuition. As you embark on this new phase of your life, you are going to need all four of those things! In addition, you will benefit from the experience of spaciousness that meditation allows you to practice. Remember, it's all about practicing the new habits that you want to create in your life!

The Three Types of Meditation

I often find when my clients come to me that they are already using guided meditations. There are so many great resources for guided meditation in the world, and I'm delighted that it's becoming so accessible for people. However, my recommendation is always to work towards having the meditation in your practice be under your own guidance. Meditating under your own guidance forces you to learn how to take control of your own mind which is a skill you must learn in order to do this work. It also creates a space where you can be more available to receive your own guidance.

The style of meditation I teach does not derive from any one specific lineage, but rather distills the major schools of meditation into three basic disciplines.

The first type of meditation is a concentration, or focus, meditation. In a concentration meditation, you choose one point of focus to hold your mind on. This may be a mantra or a single candle flame. A very common way to begin is to simply count your breaths backward from ten like this:

Inhale – ten –
Exhale – nine –
Inhale – eight –
Exhale – seven –

…and so on. Allow a brief pause between each breath so your pace stays calm and mindful.

You can also focus on a single candle flame or an affirmation such as "peace" or "love."

This is the type of meditation that I recommend most people begin with. I suggest adding a ten-minute focus meditation following your writing for the second week of your practice.

The second type of meditation is an awareness, or insight, meditation. In awareness meditation there is no technique. You simply observe.

One of my teachers describes it like this: "Imagine that your mind is a movie screen, and your thoughts are a movie playing on the screen. Every time you see a thought on the screen, point at it and say 'thought.' Let the thoughts come and go without trying to stop or change them."

You might also simply watch your breath or be aware of the sensations in your body.

I often find this type of meditation is trickier for beginners. It is a great way to become aware of your thoughts and notice your thought patterns, but it can be easy to get caught up in your thoughts and just spend your whole meditation time thinking.

I recommend adding ten minutes of this technique *after* your concentration meditation. So now your practice looks like: stream-of-consciousness writing, concentration meditation, awareness meditation. Do this after you've already been practicing the concentration meditation for a week or so. Don't get frustrated if your mind wanders or you get caught up in your thoughts. Just notice that it's happened and then go back to watching the thoughts. The course correction is just as important to practice as the actual state of meditation.

The third type of meditation is visualization. The Cabin meditation is a visualization style of meditation. In visualization, you may be visualizing a place, an intention, or a state of being. You will also incorporate visualization more into your practice when we get to Chapter 8.

To begin with, practice your stream of consciousness writing, your concentration meditation, and your awareness meditation. These will give you the tools you need to really become skilled at making powerful choices further along in the process.

But I Can't Meditate!

I frequently hear from people that they can't meditate because they can't clear their minds. To me, that's akin to someone who has never done weightlifting saying that they can't exercise because they can't bench press 500 pounds.

What I teach is that it's not the purpose of meditation to clear your mind. It's the purpose of meditation for you to work with your mind, to increase the capacity of what your mind is capable of just like exercise increases the capacity of what your body is capable of. Concentration meditation strengthens your ability to focus; awareness meditation allows you to draw new insights and connections in your life. These are practiced skills.

With time, a regular meditation practice does lead to a clearer mind, and this is a great benefit. But when you are in meditation, there is no need to keep trying to clear your mind. Thoughts will arise. That's what the mind does: it thinks. You let the thoughts be. They will arise, one will follow on the next. Your job in meditation is just to notice those thoughts and then to bring your attention back to the meditation technique that you are practicing.

Imagine being in a room with a bunch of noisy kids running all over the place. The way we often interact with our thoughts is like running after the kids all day. When you meditate, you learn how to sit quietly in the middle of the room. The kids are still running around and being wild, but you aren't bothered by them anymore, and you definitely aren't chasing them.

And the magic is, if you sit calmly for long enough then eventually the kids will notice, and they will come sit calmly with you. The same thing will happen with your thoughts. If you let them be then eventually they will calm down on their own.

But I Can't Sit Still!

A lot of times when people start meditating they struggle to sit still for long periods of time. It is so important to be compassionate with yourself about this! In the beginning, it will be hard to sit in meditation. This requires some discipline like we discussed earlier. But it's also so important that you find ways to enjoy your meditation! If your meditation always feels hard, then you will never want to do it. Your brain will actually find ways to make it harder to do, and you won't succeed in your practice.

The first thing you need to do in order to have a successful practice is to find a way to make it enjoyable, even if it is also challenging. The brain likes to be challenged, but it doesn't like to be punished. On a neurological level, you are setting yourself up for more success with your practice and with the changes you are making in your life if you can find a way to make your practice enjoyable.

Here are three ways to make your practice more enjoyable:

1. **Create sacred space:** Making a special place where you always go for your practice can help remind you that this is a supportive ritual you are creating for yourself. This does not have to be a spartan monk's cell. My meditation space is full of little things that remind me to take delight in life—crystals, inspiring pictures, bottles of essences, little toys. Even if you don't have a big space to carve out, what could you put in your sacred space that would help inspire your practice?

2. **You don't have to sit still:** This is a common misconception about meditation. You don't actually have to sit still, and you definitely don't have to twist yourself into a pretzel. You can meditate sitting in a chair; you can meditate lying down; you can meditate standing; you can meditate with your eyes closed; you can meditate with your eyes open; you can meditate while walking; you can meditate while singing; you can meditate while dancing or shaking or crying. To meditate with movement, you can choose an intention and keep your mind on that intention

as you move. For example, as you sweep the floor you might hold the intention that you are sweeping away what is no longer needed in your life. Or you can practice mindfulness meditation as you move and simply stay very aware of the feelings in your body, noticing the sensations and noticing how your body feels as it moves through space. For example, if you are walking, then you might notice the pace of your steps, how your foot lands on the earth. You might also become very aware or your surroundings—the quality of the light, the temperature of the air, what you see.

3. **Reward yourself:** Especially in the beginning of your practice, accountability is key. When I first started meditating, I created a spreadsheet with my coach. We agreed on my goals for meditation, and I tracked them every day. I found that having the outside accountability of my coach and spreadsheet made it much easier to keep my commitment to myself. And then when I did it, I had a special reward planned to celebrate my accomplishment.

When Should I Stop My Practice?

Once you start your practice, you will see shifts naturally start to happen in your life. You will start to see where you have other choices available to you. Your days may start to feel easier. You may have more energy. These practices are naturally healing, and you will start to enjoy the benefits of that.

Often, I see that people use this as an excuse to stop their practice. In fact, there are three main reasons I see why people stop in their practice:

1. **Everything is going well:** The logic here is that things have gotten so much better, so I probably don't need my practice any more. What this fails to take into account is that the reason why things got better is that you did the practice. Don't use this as a reason to stop!

2. **Everything is going terribly:** The logic here is that everything is just too crazy right now, so I can't make time for my practice. What this doesn't acknowledge is that your practice can help you get the craziness under control. Don't use this as a reason to stop!

3. **Nothing is happening:** Plateaus are a natural part of life. When it feels like everything is pretty much going along fine, it's easy to feel like you don't need your practice any more. In my experience, plateaus are one of two things—you are either resting from the last big leap you took in which case your practice will help you process and integrate the lessons of that leap, or you are in incubation for your next big leap in which case it's a great time to strengthen your practice so it is there for you

when things get crazy again. Don't use this as a reason to stop!

I've known many crisis meditators (and have been one myself), and I've come to realize now that everything goes more smoothly, and I suffer so much less, if I just keep up with my practice. There is a saying, "Protect your practice, and it will protect you." I recommend making this a new mantra for yourself.

If you can learn to make your meditation and writing practice a friend and a partner, then it can see you through to a whole new way of life.

The other reason why this practice matters so much is that it gives you a space to actively refill your own well. Taking this kind of time for yourself is naturally healing. It naturally allows you to begin replenishing your own energy.

It also gives you space to see your own patterns which allows you to begin changing them.

Three Healing Practices

I want to give you three more practices specifically to help you replenish your own energy. You can add these to your morning practice or put them at the time of day when you feel most depleted. These practices are especially helpful at the end of your day to help replenish your energy. For the first two practices, I must credit my teacher Sura Kim. The third practice is my own creation.

The first practice is a grounding practice. It allows you to release energy that you've taken on from others and restore your own energy. Healers are often highly empathic, and it is easy for us to take on energy and beliefs from other people and to give away our own energy. The energy and beliefs that we take on from others can cause interference when we make choices for ourselves. It's important to release these beliefs so we can move into a new space from a place of clarity within ourselves, and it's important to be fully replenished in our own energy so we can create from a full well.

To do this practice, find an upright seated position with your feet flat on the floor. Bring all of your attention to the soles of your feet. Notice the contact points of your feet on the floor. Imagine that the floor gets softer, like soft mud, and your feet sink down into it. Visualize your legs hanging down off of the chair, and feel the weight of the bones. Imagine roots growing down from your legs, deep into the earth. See yourself releasing other people, other situations, any beliefs or expectations, any tension, the past, and the future down through the roots into the earth. Feel the sensation in your body as you easily let go, releasing everything that doesn't exist for you in present moment without any effort. Notice what it feels like to be completely grounded and present in your body.

The second practice allows you to recall and refresh your energy. You can move into this practice directly from your grounding practice. For this practice, envision a golden sun above the crown of your head, and set the intention of lovingly calling your all of your own energy back to the golden sun. You can see it coming back from clients, from coworkers, from your family, from situations in the past, and from things that you may be worrying about or anticipating in the future. As your energy returns, see the golden sun get brighter, and feel the warmth of it. When you feel that the golden sun is fully charged up, bring it down through your crown, through your neck, your chest, your belly, and all the way to the base of your spine. Feel the golden light expand through your whole body, all the way out to your fingertips and toes. Even feel it extend beyond the boundaries of your physical body until you are sitting in a golden orb full of your own energy. Notice what it feels like to sit entirely filled with your own energy. Notice the quality of it. Notice if it has a shape or color. Breathe it in, and allow it to fully permeate your whole body. Bring in as many golden suns as you need to feel fully refreshed and nourished.

The third practice allows you to center your energy. I often find that when my clients are moving in a new direction (and yes, it happens to me too!), their energy vacillates between big excitement/expansion and fear/contraction. This practice allows you to shift into a place of centered energy, which is much more sustainable and also allows for much clearer decision-making. You can link this practice directly after the golden suns practice.

For this practice, sit forward away from your seat back a little bit so you can move. Connect back in with your sense of grounding first. And then feel your head float upward so your spine gets pulled gently long without any strain or effort. Begin to take a small lean forward and backward, keeping your spine long so you don't bend at the waist. This movement can be very small, just enough to feel a weight shift. Notice what part of your body leads the movement. Is it your head? Your chest? Or does the movement initiate all the way at the base of the spine? When we get off center, it often feels like the head or the chest are leading more. If you notice that happening, then visualize allowing your center of gravity to drop slowly through the center of your body all the way to the base of your spine. You can see this happening like the ball dropping on New Year's Eve. As you see your center of gravity drop, feel how your head, your heart, and your belly all move together with balanced effort. Once this feeling is calm and even, bring it to stillness in the center and feel yourself resting right in the center of your body— neither advancing nor retreating.

Make a habit of cultivating this grounded, centered space in your body, fully inhabiting your own energy. This is a great place to make decisions from and is also very restorative for your energy.

The Heart Walk

The final practice I will offer you in this chapter is the Heart Walk. The Heart Walk is a practice that I developed to help myself become faster at tapping into and following the messages from my heart and intuition. The practice is simple. Intentionally set aside a block of time when you have nowhere to be and nothing to do. During this time, just notice what impulses arise and follow them.

This started for me with going for a walk or a drive, and every time I got to an intersection, I would just notice which direction I felt drawn toward and then turn that way. But you don't actually have to be in motion. You might get the impulse to stay home and color. You might get the impulse to sit and look out the window for an hour.

It doesn't matter what you do—and it may seem a little silly. What matters is that you listen and follow what you hear. This is a kind of playdate for your heart. It gives you a chance to practice the skills of listening, noticing, and trusting what you hear from your heart and then putting that into action. It may feel like a diversion, but this is at the heart (pardon my pun!) of what we are doing with this work. This is a practice that helps to unlock synchronicities and more ease in any other changes that you are making.

As you practice, things in your life will start to enter more of a flow state, change will naturally start to bubble up, and that will put you right into position for the topic that we cover in our next chapter: resistance!

CHAPTER 7

RESISTANCE IS FUTILE

When you start making changes, you are going to encounter resistance. Resistance is the collection of all the internal devices that your own mind and body use to keep you from making changes. It will sound like excuses; it will look like drama or distractions or feel overwhelming; it will appear to be very logical reasons why you shouldn't be doing any of the things you are doing; it will feel super uncomfortable; it may even be painful. If you listen closely, no matter how it shows up, the message from resistance will be that you should go back to how things were before.

How you meet resistance will determine your success. And I want to let you know right now that you can actually make this as fun or as hard as you want to. It's completely up to you.

If you are a nerd like me, you may remember the Borg from *Star Trek*. The Borg were a super powerful alien race that took over other races and made them into more Borg. The motto of the Borg was, "Resistance is futile."

I know a lot of people who approach resistance with a "resistance is futile" attitude. When they feel resistance, they strengthen their resolve, they get more determined, and they push through toward their goal.

Here's the problem with this: Resistance is a part of you. It is created by your own subconscious mind, and it is coming from inside of you. So, think about this—if you get stronger and push harder with your own energy, what is going to happen to this resistance that is also a part of you? It's just going to get stronger and push back harder! Resistance is always as strong as you are because it is you!

You cannot outmuscle resistance. It just gets stronger with you.

Fortunately, you don't have to! There is another way to work with resistance. It's way more effective, and it's way more fun too.

Making Resistance Your Friend

Let's pause for a moment so we can understand resistance a little better. Where does this mysterious force that seems to stand determinedly between you and accomplishing your dreams and goals really come from? Why would a part of you want to stop this process from happening?

The reason resistance shows up is actually to keep us safe. It's a survival mechanism. Resistance comes from the part of your mind tasked with making sure that you survive. What that part of your mind sees is that you have survived up to this point in your life, so what you are doing must be working. Therefore, it is safest to keep doing exactly what you are doing now.

If you think about it from that perspective, it makes a lot of sense that a part of you would resist change. There is no way to know that change is safe. So, a part of what our resistance is telling us is, "Don't change." But if we listen carefully, then there will be a more nuanced message which will sound more like, "If you are going to change, then make sure you keep these important things in mind in order to be safe."

I think of this a bit like my mom. My mom definitely has my best interest at heart, and she just wants me to be happy. But listen, I'm an ambitious gal who likes to explore and do big things in her life. I think that's a little scary for my mom sometimes. She wants me to accomplish my dreams and goals, but she also doesn't want me to get hurt. So, she'll give me advice that she hopes will keep me safe. Sometimes, although it is meant in only a loving way, the advice that she gives me may also keep me from growing. (I'm sure she'll read this, so, hi Mom! I love you, and I'm super grateful that you are always trying to do what you think is best for me!) For a time in my life, I resisted listening to any of her advice so I wouldn't have to hear the parts that would keep me from growing. But over time, I've learned how to hear the parts that could help to keep me safe while still staying committed to my own growth.

Resistance is like this. It's always trying to tell us something, and when we stop and listen, we can learn a lot. Resistance may actually be trying to give us the key we need to the next step of our growth. But we have to stop and really listen to it in order to sort through the parts of the resistance that come from fear and the parts that have real insight.

CLARA

There is a method that I learned in studying peaceful conflict resolution that I've found applies so well to resistance. It's called CLARA. The letters stand for Center, Listen, Affirm, Respond, and Add Information. Approaching resistance in this way reframes it from something that is trying to stop you to something that is trying to help you.

When using this method, it helps to use a visualization meditation to picture your resistance as a person. To do this, first get grounded and centered (use the centering techniques from the last chapter to help with this), and acknowledge that you are in resistance. Then, ask a representative to step forward and talk to you about it. With practice, you may discover that you have a whole host of different people representing your resistance. When you see which character shows up, you'll immediately have a clue about what the resistance is about.

I have a guy named Bob with a shotgun who shows up when I'm feeling really vulnerable. I have a gal named Molly who drives a car and just wants to make sure we follow the rules of the road. She shows up when things are feeling out of control. I have a lawyer who hasn't told me her name yet, but she is a super sharp dresser, and she shows up to present logical concerns with what I've proposed.

You can allow your imagination to get involved here and be playful. This is a part of how you can choose to make this process more fun for yourself.

Whether you imagine your resistance as a person or not, you need to first ground and center yourself (you can use the practices from the last chapter to help with that), and then address the resistance directly. Invite it to tell you what its concerns are, and really listen.

This is so key! You have to listen to what it tells you and also the real fears underneath what it's saying. It might say, "Well if you do this, then everyone is going to think you are so selfish, and maybe you are selfish, and if you are selfish then, that means you're a bad person, and if you're a bad person, then you can't be a healer, so clearly this is all a terrible idea."

This is the point where I think it's so helpful to imagine your resistance as another person because it gives you a little space or detachment from what the resistance is telling you. If you can maintain a little detachment, then you can just get really curious about what you are hearing.

Curiosity might sound like, "People are going to think I'm selfish? Who is going to think I'm selfish? Why does that matter? Is it really true that I'm being selfish?"

Just ask questions and really listen to the responses. This is all the "Listen" part of the process.

After you listen for a bit, you'll start to sort out which aspects of the resistance are useful and which are based in old beliefs or old ways of being that you aren't choosing any more.

Once you can start to see that, then it will be easier to shift into gratitude for the ways that your resistance is trying to keep you safe. This is the "Affirm" step. It might sound something like this: "Wow, thank you for bringing all of that to my attention. I hear you. I really appreciate how you are looking out for me and how you always have my back. There is really no one else in my life who is so committed to keeping me safe as you are. What I'm hearing that's really important here is…"

I know that may sound hokey, but try it! There is no faster way to shift resistance than to genuinely thank it for showing up. You will feel the effect immediately. If you don't feel a shift, then you haven't truly heard what it has to tell you yet. Remember, the point of this isn't to make the resistance go away; the point is to learn what useful information the resistance has for you. If you haven't done that yet, then you won't feel a shift at this point. Go back to listening some more.

Once you feel the shift, then you are free to respond specifically to the points that came up. You can say, "I know you are really worried about what Jane will think of me if I make this change. After talking to you, I've realized that it is a good idea to have a conversation with her so she isn't blindsided by the new things that I'm doing. Thank you for bringing that to my attention."

And then, only after you've done all of that, you can add more information. You might say, "I know this may seem really selfish, and according to my old-world view, it would have been. But what I've realized is that in order to be my best self and offer my greatest service to the world, I need to take better care of myself. So that is why I'm making these new choices. I hope you'll be able to help me keep making these choices that allow me to show up as a more refreshed and fuller version of myself."

What I think happens most of the time when people meet resistance is they go straight to the last step—they try to tell the resistance, "Listen, this is the new direction; just get on board with me!" without taking the in-between steps.

The in-between steps are where the gold is! That's where you get to find out what this part of you that really, *really* wants to keep you safe is trying to tell you. Don't skip those steps! It may seem counterintuitive, but the faster you can turn toward your resistance, the faster and more easily you'll be able to move forward in your life.

I used to spend days, weeks, even months wrestling with my resistance. At this point in my life, if I notice that I'm dealing with the same resistance for even a couple of hours, I make time to work with it. If it lasts more than a day or if I'm not able to hear what it has to tell me, I bring it to my coach. There is just way too much value in that information to miss out on what it has to tell me.

What Thought Will You Have?

As you deepen in your own practice, you will start to become more aware of how to separate your thoughts from your circumstances. For example, if you have a circumstance where you realize that you've taken on more than you can sustainably manage, you might have the thought, "I can't believe I let people walk all over me like this!"

The thought is neither true nor untrue; it's just what you are thinking about the circumstance. Another thought you could have in the same situation is, "Oh, here's a good opportunity for me to practice bringing my life into better balance. I wonder what step I could take to get started on that."

Really start to watch your thoughts and what stories you tell yourself about your circumstances. When you do this, you can actually start to choose the thoughts that will move you forward.

It helps to choose one or two go-to thoughts for when challenging situations arise so you can reach for your thought right away before you get stuck in telling yourself stories about the circumstance. It's important to do this in advance because by the time you are feeling super uncomfortable, it's already too late.

And you will have times when you feel super uncomfortable. It just comes with making change.

Start to notice what you tell yourself about your discomfort when it arises. For example, if you're holding a new boundary that requires you to say no when in the past you would have said yes, then that will generally feel quite uncomfortable. Or if you decide that you need to raise your rates, then that will often feel quite uncomfortable in the beginning.

Notice what you say to yourself in that moment of discomfort. Do you tell yourself that this means you've made a wrong decision? Do you tell yourself that your discomfort means that this isn't going to work?

The reality is that discomfort is a very normal, natural, and even healthy part of change. There is nothing fundamentally wrong with feeling discomfort when you make a change. Except of course the no one likes to be uncomfortable. I get it—I don't like it either.

So a part of this process is normalizing that discomfort for yourself, and this is where choosing your thought in advance is really helpful. Here are a few thoughts that I've found helpful:

- This is just what change feels like, and it's totally normal.
- Everything that shows up in this process is here to help me move forward in it, even my discomfort.
- As long as I keep showing up, I know I can make progress on my goals.
- If I get through this uncomfortable thing now, then later I will offer myself the gift of…
- This feels awful right now, but the reason why it is important is…

Choose a thought that helps you reconnect to your motivation or inspiration. It needs to be a thought that you believe a least as much as a thought that you are replacing. Something that you can reach for quickly as soon as you notice the discomfort starting to arise. I recommend writing your thought on a sticky note and posting it in a place that you will see regularly. This can help you ride the waves of discomfort without getting pulled under into negative stories or old beliefs.

The Gift of Anger

One of your tasks in this work is to become a ninja at identifying different kinds of discomfort. As you begin to move through the layers of change, you will experience many kinds of discomfort, and if you can identify the type of discomfort, then you can more appropriately address it.

Some discomfort comes from resistance as we discussed earlier. This needs to be addressed internally and listened to.

Some discomfort comes as a natural part of making change. A lot of this is the natural grief of releasing the person you used to be as the new you is brought forth. You can address this discomfort by being really kind and gentle with yourself, practicing good self-care, and bringing your mind back to the thought you chose above.

Some discomfort comes when you take on other people's energy. You can address this discomfort by using your grounding and golden suns practice in the last chapter to clear and restore your own energy.

With practice, you will be able to quickly identify which type of discomfort you are feeling and know how to best address it. But there is one more major type of discomfort that we haven't identified yet, and that is anger.

Anger can feel like healer kryptonite.

As caring people, it can feel like we are not allowed to own or even feel our anger. I pushed away my own anger and resentment for years. When I did try to express it, I was often met with shame and rebuke. It felt much safer to just show a happy face to the world, even when I was suffering on the inside.

But anger is a powerful teacher; it will show you where you are out of integrity if you listen. You must find a constructive way to work with it.

What is the message of anger? Anger shows us when a boundary has been crossed. Resentment is often the tip-of-the-iceberg version of anger. It may feel unsafe to allow yourself to know how angry you truly are, so you can only allow yourself to feel resentment. Pay attention to your resentments! They may be masking much deeper issues.

Why does all of this matter so much to you as a healer? Well, remember that healing work is heart work. You can probably feel the truth of that in your body. When you feel truly connected to someone, when you can both feel that real healing is happening, you will feel it in your heart.

And the foundation of heart work is compassion. The journey toward creating balance in your life will require that you have enormous compassion for yourself. And one block to that compassion is anger.

Brené Brown says this well in her book *The Gifts of Imperfection*: "The better we are at accepting ourselves, the more compassionate we become. Well, it's difficult to accept people when they are hurting us or taking advantage of us or walking all over us. [The] research has told me that if we really want to practice compassion, we have to start by setting boundaries and holding people accountable for their behavior."

Read that a couple of times. Take it in. Because what it's saying is that in order to effectively do healing work (which is heart work, which is compassion work) we must actually turn toward our anger and acknowledge where we are being taken advantage of.

And at this point, the resentments can rise, and it can feel oh-so-tempting to blame other people—our clients, our patients, our spouses, our kids, our parents—to say that other people are the ones who are taking advantage of us, hurting us, walking all over us.

That's the shadow side of the martyr mentality.

See it. Recognize it. Love yourself even when it comes up. We all do it—me too.

But the healing comes when you realize that not one of those other people you might want to point the finger at is the one who is allowing the situation in this present moment. The only person who can allow your boundaries to be crossed, my dear, and I say this with all love and empathy because I've done it too, is you.

And that is the gift of anger. Anger shows you where you are accepting situations that aren't actually acceptable to you.

Do the work with your anger, yes. Listen to it, do your grounding, do your meditation. But be aware that anger doesn't go away unless you address the situation that created it. Anger will always show you where you need to take action.

That's why it's such a hot, driving, uncomfortable feeling. It feels that way so you won't be able to ignore it.

When you get to this point in your journey, you may have a difficult reckoning because what you realize is that the person you are actually angry with is yourself—for allowing the situation and for allowing people to cross your boundaries.

This is a time for extreme gentleness. Give yourself time to rest, space to heal. Explore how you can offer yourself forgiveness. Strengthen your daily practice.

Your emotions may be all over the place. That's okay. Keep breathing. This is what it feels like to unlock a piece of yourself that you've shut away and tried not to look at.

I promise that you will make it through this stage, and things will feel better again.

If at all possible, I recommend waiting to take those actions and having the conversations about those boundaries until you've taken some space for your own inner healing. You will come from a much clearer space and suffer less through the new boundaries if you can find your way through to forgive yourself before taking big actions in the world.

One of the most important tools I know during this time is to keep reaching out for help to people who you know and trust to have an empathetic response.

As healers and caregivers, we are so often taught that anger is a shameful emotion. If shame gets its hooks in you, then this stage will last much, much longer than it needs to and can cause significant trauma.

I had an experience of this on my own path to thriving that I want to share with you so you can see what happens. As I was doing my own work, I realized that my relationship with my first business partner was extremely unhealthy. It took me a long time to see how truly toxic this situation was for me, but once I saw it, I very quickly made the decision to end it. I didn't have the time to do my own healing or forgiveness work first, and I didn't have my own practice in place at the time.

As a result of ending the partnership, a lot of people were very angry with me. They told me what a terrible person I was, how selfish I was being. It felt like all of my worst fears realized.

Lacking a personal practice and not having done any self-forgiveness work in advance, I started to believe them. I started to feel ashamed of what I'd done and believe that it was wrong, even though I knew deep-down that it wasn't. I felt like I couldn't talk to anyone about my true experience.

I spent a long time in very harsh judgement of myself which led me to make other choices that also didn't respect my own boundaries. It took an incredible amount of work for me to feel safe again and secure in the knowledge that I'd made a necessary choice for my own health and life.

I do not want you to have to walk through that dark place if I can prevent it. This is why I offer you the tools of your personal practice, doing your own healing work, and reaching out for help.

Brené Brown says, "Shame hates it when we reach out and tell our story. It hates having words wrapped around it—it can't stand being shared. Shame loves secrecy. The most dangerous thing to do after a shaming experience is to hide or bury our story. When we bury our story, the shame metastasizes."

If you find that your healer recovery leads you into these murky waters, please find the people in your inner circle—a coach, friends, a counsellor, a spouse—who can hear your whole story with empathy and hold that healing space for you.

This will be hugely helpful to keep you moving forward.

There is a natural process of alignment that will start to unfold as you use the tools we've already explored. In a body, alignment happens when all of the different body parts work together in a harmonious and efficient way. In a life and a business, alignment is the same. You experience alignment when your thoughts, your beliefs, and your values are all in harmony with your actions.

You create greater alignment by taking aligned actions. That may sound obvious, but I see people get stuck at this stage so often. They don't want to move forward or make changes until they figure out what they need to do in order to take just the right action.

This is the stage where you need to give yourself permission to let things get messy. You will never get into alignment just in your own head. Alignment comes from taking aligned action which means making changes in your life.

Using the tools I've taught you so far may help you to feel better in your life as it is right now, but I just want to make it really clear that my purpose here isn't to help you feel better. My purpose is to free you to create your life in a way that is actually sustainable, joyful, and spacious for you. You'll probably discover along the way that in order to come into sustainable alignment you need to make some changes. A few changes that my clients have discovered they need to make in order to get themselves into alignment include: decreasing the number of hours that they spend with clients, raising their rates, hiring someone to help them with their work, or changing the work that they are doing.

This is the work of moving FORWARD!

Putting it All Together

The FORWARD method is an approach that I developed for accessing and acting on intuition. It incorporates all the skills you've learned so far into one tool that you can use any time you start to feel stuck or need to make a choice. You can also use this approach for your meditation in your daily practice. I find that it offers instant clarity and puts you directly into a state where you are prepared to take aligned actions.

Use this method any time you are stuck, you have a question, or you simply need to shift your state of being. In the beginning, you will probably need to carve out the space to practice this method as a full meditation. It can become the meditation half of your daily practice. As you become more skillful, you'll be able to do this at any time in your life without missing a beat.

Focus: The first step is to focus your awareness on an intention, an inspiration, a state of being, or a question. Your practice with concentration meditation will pay off here. One of my teachers says, "the state that you are sitting in is the state that you create," and I find this so applicable in every area of life. If you find yourself in a contracted state, a state of fear, in worry, or in doubt then that is what you will focus on. By bringing your focus back to your inspiration or an expansive question, you will instantly start to shift your awareness into a space where you are more able to notice more possibilities.

Open your awareness: The next step is to make some space around your point of focus. If you are asking a question, just allow it to be a question without grasping at an answer. If you are focusing on an inspiration or a state of being, then just give it space to be and expand. Imagine how it is to be with someone that you feel so comfortable around them that you can both sit in silence and still feel connected to one another. That is the feeling here. Just be with your point of focus and give it space. Your awareness meditation practice will really help with this step.

Relax: As you maintain your focus and open your awareness around it, allow your body to relax. Visualize your shoulders melting down away from your ears. Allow yourself to take a deep breath. Check your hands, feet, and face, and let go of any muscles you are holding. If your eyes are open, soften your vision. Allow yourself to ground and center yourself in your body. This is like the step of listening in the CLARA method and opens you up to receive insight.

What do you notice? Just like in CLARA, be curious and open. Observe what arises and bubbles up. Pay special attention to how your heart feels as you meditate on questions or different options, and notice the first moment of response. Does it feel expansive and open or squeezed and constricted? What else do you notice? You may notice resistance; you may hear words or messages; you may notice a feeling or an emotion; you may see images. Just observe. Make it a game to see how many things you can notice.

Allow it to be OK: Whatever comes up, allow it to be OK without judgement. When you go into judgement, you actually use a different part of your brain that shuts down your ability to learn, so actively shifting into allowance creates a space where it is possible to learn and grow. If you notice resistance or an uncomfortable feeling, you may need to pause and use CLARA to work with the resistance. Just play with the space of allowance.

Receive guidance: This entire process helps you to create a state of consciousness where you can receive guidance.

How you view this guidance depends on your world view. You may see it as intuition or divine guidance or simply insight. For my purposes, it doesn't matter how you label it. What matters is that you tune into it. This is where you will start to see the paths that are aligned for you, gain insight, and receive answers to your questions. Continue tuning into your heart in this process. Notice what draws you in, what feels light, what stimulates your curiosity. In this process, you don't choose your work; it chooses you.

Decide and trust: This is where you move your insights and guidance into action. It's important to notice that this step says, "decide and trust" and not just "trust." I did that not only because FORWART isn't as memorable as FORWARD but also because at this point you must make an active choice about how you will take action on your guidance and then also make the decision to trust your choice. Trust always has to be a choice. There will be times when your guidance points you toward a course that feels super uncomfortable or doesn't seem to make any sense. You always have the choice about whether or not you follow the guidance, but either way, make it an active choice. Don't just trust; *decide* that you are going to trust, and then, take action. If you decide not to follow the guidance, make that an active choice and then decide to trust your choice. This is a key to keep you out of victim mindset. If you decide to trust then you are moving forward in an empowered way and if things don't work out the way you'd thought, then you'll be in a more active place to say, "Ok, things are sticky now, but I made this decision because I trusted my guidance. I wonder what the guidance is for moving FORWARD from here?" And then you can step right back into the process.

CHAPTER 9

A BUSY LIFE
VS. A FULL LIFE

The work we've been doing up to this point is mostly inner work. What I've found is that this inner work is necessary in order to actually take the action steps that create alignment between mind, body, and spirit. You now have the tools you need to transform your life.

The question now is just how to put them into action. In order have a new experience, you're going to need to take new actions.

At this point, my clients have usually started to realize what changes they need to make in their lives, and they also often start to tell me about why they can't make those changes. A few common reasons why include: I don't have the time; I don't have the money; it's just not what I do. All of these reasons are cover-ups for deeper issues.

I want you to stop accepting these excuses from yourself. For example, if you accept the excuse that you are too busy, then that means that you are not in control of your own schedule and life, and you are not willing to take responsibility for the choice of how you spend your time.

You may choose to have an intentionally full life—I fill my life with work that I love and time with my husband and ambitious projects and travel and time with my dogs because I love all of those things, and I choose to have them all in my life. But notice the difference between that energy of choosing to have a full life versus the energy of being too busy to do the things you want to do. This is another subtle shift out of victim mindset.

My client Susan, who was transitioning into a coaching business from a full-time job as a physician's assistant, ran into this block with building her business. She felt like she was just too busy to give it the time it needed. I told her, "Well OK, you're too busy, but if you could make time to work on your business, when would it be?"

After thinking for a while, she realized she could take some time on the weekends. It would mean cutting family time shorter, but she could do it.

Then I challenged her again: "Ok, when else could you make time?"

She realized she could bring her lunch to work and do work on her business over her lunch hour.

"Great," I said, "when else could you make time?"

She admitted that she could carve out an hour in the evenings after her kids went to bed.

"Ok, I bet you can find another bit of time," I prompted.

And then she remembered that she had a lot of unused vacation time that she could take to work on her business as well.

In the span of about fifteen minutes, Susan went from having no time to work on her business to having four different options of time to work on her business! With a little more coaching, she realized that taking vacation time to work on her business felt like the best option for her energy, and that's when we discovered her real resistance to making time for her business.

"It feels so selfish, taking vacation time for my own business. If I'm taking time off, I feel like I should be spending it with my children!" she said.

Bingo! She'd been using the excuse "I'm too busy," but what she really meant was, "I feel guilty spending time on something for myself." Once she made that realization, we were able to do some coaching around that guilt, and she suddenly had plenty of time to work on her business.

The one time when I will say that you are allowed to use the "I'm too busy" excuse is with other people, so long as you do it mindfully. People respect the excuse "I'm too busy to do that right now," and it may be more tactful than saying "I'm choosing not to go to your party because I just don't prioritize it very highly right now." Use your own judgement on this one! Just don't use the excuse with yourself.

Go Fast!

Another belief that a lot of my clients hold is that it needs to take a long time to transform your business. Again, this is a form of resistance that gives you an excuse to stay where you are. Don't accept this excuse from yourself.

In fact, find a reason why you need to go fast. What will your motivation be? My clients who can afford to move slowly through this transition do, and they end up spending a lot longer in the uncomfortable parts of the transition. My clients who have a reason why they need to move fast blow even me away with how quickly they can move. I will give you two examples.

I will use myself as the example of how to do this the painful way, so I don't need to pick on any of my clients. A few years back, before I had learned that you can make these things as easy or as painful as you want to, I realized that I was teaching way too much and burning myself out. I knew I needed to cut my hours, but I also knew I needed to raise my rates to cover the difference in the hours I would be working. On top of that, I was having a problem where a lot of my clients were being really inconsistent with their lessons—one client took nearly a year to use one ten-pack of lessons— which meant that they weren't getting great results, and that was another source of burnout for me. So, I knew that I not only needed to change my rates but also the structure of how I billed my clients so they would show up consistently for their lessons.

I knew (or I decided) this was going to be really difficult. I decided people weren't going to like my new schedule and rates, and I was going to have to figure out how to do it just right. I decided I would take as much time as I needed to in order to get this transition right.

Ten months, and so, so, *so* much suffering later, I had finally transitioned to my new schedule and business model. I spent months obsessing over exactly what timing I wanted for the transition and how to tell people and whether it was going to work and worrying that it wouldn't, but in the end, I was still making a living, the sky hadn't fallen, and everything was fine.

Compare this to my client Jennifer.

Jennifer came to me because she desperately needed to get out of her job. Her boss was borderline emotionally abusive, her long commute was making her sick, and as a result of her high stress level, her marriage was falling apart.

As a physical therapist, Jennifer loved working with her patients, and she'd even developed her own method for a specific kind of injury recovery that was having great success. She wanted to have her own business so she could maintain ownership of the method she'd developed and use it to serve a lot more patients in an environment that was healthy for her.

Jennifer's situation gave her the impetus she needed to move fast. Within two months of beginning our work together, Jennifer had found an investor, developed a business plan, and was in the process of opening a new clinic where she would be in charge. It was an amazing amount of change in a very short period of time, but it worked because Jennifer just calmly asked at each step, "Ok, what next?"

The key here is in letting go of the expectation of perfection. You let go of perfection by insistently asking yourself the question, "How can I best serve myself and the people that I'm on this planet to serve with what is available to me *right now*?"

I've learned that I can apply this lesson in any area of life. I only commit to things that really matter, that are a clear yes for me at that time, and then I have the impetus I need to move fast and improve as I go so I don't spend a lot of time suffering in the "got to get it right" land of perfectionism.

I see that this mindset makes a huge difference in my clients' success and also how they feel along the way.

Reframe Clarity

Most people assume that clarity means knowing where you are going to end up. This is another place where I see people get stuck so often. It can come with various names. I often hear people saying they just need to brainstorm or do more research. It generally feels like you need to know where you are going or where you plan to end up before you can get started.

This is a very logical thought, but it can also easily become a block.

What clarity actually means is just knowing what step to take next. The larger vision comes into focus only after you've started moving which requires trusting your guidance and getting started.

This does feel scary—I completely acknowledge that! But it is also a how any heart-centered journey looks. Even though you may not know where you are going to end up, you still can get clear guidance from your heart and intuition about what step to take next and which direction to head in.

I compare it to feeling like you are falling forward, and with each step, you just trust that the next stepping stone will appear before your foot lands. This is where your practice and knowing what thought you want to have about discomfort are so critical to keep you grounded and calm as you move through the space of uncertainty and fear.

Know Your Energy

Start to observe your energy. Notice how you feel throughout the week. What clients energize you? What clients drain your energy? Notice whether there are types of work that energize you more. Just get really curious and let anything you notice be okay. All of this will help you in building a sustainable schedule for your work that serves your energy (and by extension, serves your clients).

If you notice that you are getting drained, try to do experiments to find out if it is the client, the type of work, the time of day, or some other variable that is draining you.

For example, I discovered that if I teach movement on Wednesday mornings, it drains my energy. It doesn't matter who I teach—I tried putting a number of different clients in that time slot. And I can coach on Wednesday mornings and be fine. But if I teach movement on Wednesday mornings, my energy will be drained.

I resisted that insight for a long time because it doesn't make any sense! Why would coaching on a Wednesday morning be fine, but teaching wouldn't? And why Wednesday mornings? However, once I finally just accepted it and allowed it to be okay, I was able to build my schedule in a way where I don't teach on Wednesday morning, and my energy stays much higher throughout the week.

The more you tune into these insights, the more you will see not only what hours you can work sustainably but also who you want to work with and what work you want to do with them.

Again, this comes back to connecting to your heart.

When you follow what truly speaks to your heart, you can tap into an inexhaustible and expansive flow of energy. It naturally replenishes itself as long as you are staying in the zone where you are listening and following what the heart tells you. As healers, we are often told to hold boundaries, to say "no," and when we do, that it feels constrictive. Since it doesn't feel expansive, it rings false—it doesn't match the expansive feeling of choosing from the heart. This is why healers often struggle to hold healthy boundaries.

Don't make "no" your first go-to in changing your life. Instead, pay attention to what you are saying "yes" to. The one and only secret to not burning out is to relentlessly follow and say "yes" to only those things that are naturally expansive for your heart and to allow everything else to fall away.

Clearing Your Energy

Another part of building a sustainable schedule is making sure that you have time to refresh and renew yourself throughout the week. In addition to your daily practice, remember to ground and recall your own energy throughout the day to actively release any energy you take on from clients and bring back any energy you may have given away.

I have a little ritual I do after each client. It only takes about thirty seconds, but it allows me to consciously close the session and renew my own energy. I always recommend that my clients create such a ritual for themselves as well.

Here are a few options for what you can do to reset your energy. Some will be more appropriate as you go through your day, and some will work better at the end of the day:

1. Begin each session with the intention that you will end with your energy and the client will end with their energy

2. Practice grounding, centering, and bringing in golden suns (the exercise from Chapter 6)

3. Wash your hands between sessions and visualize the water washing away any energy that doesn't belong to you

4. Light a candle at the beginning of the session and blow it out at the end of the session

5. Visualize unplugging yourself from any energy or beliefs you've taken on

6. Shake your arms and legs or stretch and yawn to help physically process any stored energy

7. Visualize sending any energy you've taken on back to its source

8. Do cross crawls (touching one hand to the opposite knee, alternating sides) to help connect the right and left brain and clear your mind

9. Do breathing exercises

10. Do a quick meditation

11. Go outside

12. Clap, shout, or make noise

13. Move or do a workout

14. Use crystals, essential oils, or other essences

15. Actively choose to step out of the healer archetype

What Do I Say?

I mentioned back in chapter three that there are several changes healers typically realize they need to make in their businesses. These include setting new boundaries around our hours or schedule, giving ourselves permission to delegate and let go of work that leaves us overextended, consistently making the space to release any energy we take on from our clients, setting our rates at a level that truly supports us, and acknowledging when it's time to move on to doing new work.

This generally leads to necessary conversations, and I find that often my clients aren't sure what to say at this point. Especially if you are still healing any old patterns within yourself that make it feel selfish to ask for what you want or need, telling clients that you can't see them anymore, that you are raising your rates, or that you won't be offering services that you used to offer can re-trigger all of those old wounds.

There are two aspects to be aware of here. The first is your own stuff. As you contemplate the conversations you need to have, notice what is getting triggered for you. What feelings arise? What stories do you have around those feelings? What do you need to do for yourself to offer healing for those triggers?

Once you can address your own triggers, then you are simply left with a messaging issue. How are you going to deliver this news in a way that acknowledges both you and the other person? Think about what the other person needs to hear and also what is the best for them in the situation.

For example, if you are telling a client you can't work with them anymore, you can say, "We've come to a point in our work where I think you'll be best served by working with another practitioner. I think this person can really help you with…"

It helps if you acknowledge for yourself that this is true—if you've realized that it isn't sustainable for your energy to work with this client, then they will be better served by working with someone else!

If they protest and say, "No, I really want to work with you!" then you can say, "I love working with you too, but I care about you too much to keep taking your money when I really think this other person will be a better fit for you. I want to give it a chance. I'll check back in, and you can let me know how it is going. If this turns out to not be the best fit, then I'll help you find another one."

Another approach is to just decide that you are going to model good boundaries and good self-care for your clients. You can be completely honest about what you are doing. For this approach you can say something like, "I want to let you know about some changes that I'm making. It's so important to me to be in integrity with the work I do, and I really can't bring my best self to my work when I'm scheduling myself the way I've been doing. So, it's been a tough decision, but I've realized I need to cut my hours back, and I won't be working at this time any more. I want to make sure you are still getting the care you need, so here are my thoughts about other options for how you can do that."

When it comes to raising your rates, I see healers make a lot of unnecessary drama about this. Prices go up in the world; it happens. People are used to it. Generally, every time I've raised my rates, my clients have said, "It's about time already!"

But I know it can feel uncomfortable, so here are a couple of ways you can message that change that have worked for me:

- **Ask for a raise.** The first time I raised my rates I wrote a letter to my clients and told them about all the training I'd done since starting my practice. I pointed out the ways I'd committed to being there for them, and I noted how long I'd been at my current rate. I then asked them for a raise to my new rates. They all agreed that I had definitely earned a raise, and there was no drama about my rate increase.

- **Increase your rates for new clients only.** If you regularly bring in new clients, you could choose to keep the same rates for your existing clients, and only raise your rates for new clients. If you choose this route, I recommend letting your existing clients know, "I'm raising my rates for new clients this fall. As a thank you for my existing clients, I'm keeping my rates the same for all of you, but I just wanted to let you know in case you refer someone to me that my rates will be a bit higher for them." With this method your current clients feel super special keeping their current rate, and even if you decide you need to raise their rates in six months, they know they still saved money for those intervening months.

- **Use it as a way to cut your hours.** If you've realized you need to cut your hours, you can do this at the same time that you raise your rates to great effect. If you tell people, "I'm cutting my hours this fall" right before you tell them, "I'm also raising my rates" then their first concern is often, "How can I stay on your schedule even when you cut your hours?" and the rate increase is less of a concern at that point. If you do have any clients who drop away as a result of your rate increase, then they will just make it that much easier to cut your hours.

Don't Neglect the Simple Stuff

As you are going through this process, don't forget about your basic needs: sleep, good nutrition, moving your body. This stuff is necessary in order to do the higher work of self-actualization.

If you start to encounter a lot of resistance or negative thinking, stop and pay attention to how much sleep you are getting, to what you've been eating. You may need more rest than usual as you start to do this work. You may need to move your body more. You may find your body needing different foods—possibly more grounding or comforting foods. As you start to shift your life, make sure to build the space in to fulfill these needs, and give yourself permission to move at a pace that allows you to continue attending to these needs.

This is a process. You won't balance your whole life overnight, but by beginning to take actions that bring your business into alignment with your own energy, you are creating a sustainable foundation for the life you truly want to be living.

CHAPTER 10

THE "M WORD"

Money is a particularly fraught subject for healers, so I'm giving it a chapter all to itself. Most healers tell me that they just aren't motivated by money which is completely valid. But there is an undercurrent that I feel/hear whenever healers start to talk about money that's something like "charging for your work pollutes the work" or "if you are really a true healer then you should be above caring about money." This is what I want to address.

Artists have a similar tendency—there's this idealized image of the "starving artist." With healers, it's more of a martyr image than a starving image, but I want us to all agree that we can move past these old beliefs about what it means to be an artist or a healer right now.

Money is how our society has chosen to handle exchanges of energy. If you are doing healing work with people, then you are offering a significant amount of your own time and energy. Charging appropriately for that service creates balance in your interactions with your clients and helps to facilitate healing.

Every overworked, out-of-balance healer I've ever worked with or encountered (including me!) has had to examine their relationship with money and how they think about charging for their services before they could balance their lives.

There is a lot of advice out there about how to charge for your services, and a lot of it will never lead to the result of having a balanced business, so let's dig right in and see what you need to be charging for your services.

Don't Charge What You Are Worth

I hear people say all the time, "I'm going to finally charge what I'm really worth!"

Don't do this! It's a terrible idea. For starters, it's not actually possible. You are priceless. There is no way to put a number on your actual worth. But if you approach how you charge for your services from this perspective, then you are telling your subconscious mind, "This number that I'm charging is how much I value myself." And at the point, your subconscious mind will always try to navigate you into situations where you feel like you are worth that amount. It becomes a self-perpetuating cycle and makes it much more difficult to raise your rates or ever make more money because on a subconscious level, you will actually resist it.

And then, when you meet people who charge more than you, your subconscious mind will say, "I'm not as valuable as those people." Which may get translated as, "I'm not as good as those people" or "I can't have as much success as those people" or something else that probably isn't true at all.

You may be able to tell that I get a little worked up about this one, but it's only because I see it lead to so many hang-ups for people that are entirely unnecessary. I love you! I don't want you to get stuck in this rut. Please don't charge what you are worth!

Don't Charge What Your Service is Worth

Okay, this is a rut I actually got stuck in for years. I knew I didn't want to charge what I was worth because it was impossible, so I said, "That's okay, I will charge what my service is worth."

But that's kind of weird, too, when you think about it. Listen, my husband is a software developer. He writes software that helps video game developers make their video games work. I'm sure that service is very valuable to the video game developers it serves, and it certainly helps them to generate a lot of money, but it still didn't seem more valuable than the service I was providing. The movement training I provide allows people to show up in their lives as happy, healthy, fully functioning members of society. It gets them out of crippling pain. My coaching work allows people to build businesses and offering healing work to so many other people.

And yet, for years, I made less money than my husband. It always made me scratch my head a little bit because if I was truly charging for the value of my service, then shouldn't I be making at least as much money as him, if not more? On an intuitive level, I felt like the service I was offering was probably of more value to the world than the one that he was offering (and he agreed, for what it's worth).

So, after years of unsuccessfully trying to make this strategy make sense to myself, I finally abandoned it.

Don't Worry About Serving Everyone

Before I tell you what I've discovered that does work, we're going to look at one more approach where I see so many healers get stuck that also doesn't work. This is the approach of pricing your services so they are accessible to everyone.

I know you are a caring person and you really want to help everyone that you can, and that can lead to pricing your services at a level that you think will be accessible to everyone. At this point, we need to pause and examine what your definition of success is in your business. What does it mean to be successful in your business? Does it mean getting as many people as possible through your door? Because if that is your measure of success, then by all means, offer very low prices.

But if you are reading this book, then I'm guessing you have a broader definition of success. A part of success probably means making a difference for as many people as possible (notice it's not the same thing to make a difference for someone as it is to get them through your door). And a part of success is also having a healthy life outside of your business.

If what I just said is closer to your definition of success, then having a lot of low-price offerings is never going to get you there. I'll explain more about why in the next section.

Charge What Will Allow You to Provide the Greatest Service

Remember when I told you in the last chapter about my client who took nearly a year to use a ten-pack of private lessons? You know why she did that? Because I told her she could get results that way. I did that with my pricing structure. At that time, my packages all had a one-year expiration date on them. Most of my clients came more frequently, but ultimately what that pricing communicated was, "If you come see me ten times in a year, then we can get some real work done together."

I thought I was doing them a favor by giving them all this time to use their package, but someone who wants to get in shape or rehab a shoulder injury or solve any of the problems that I can solve with movement is never going to see any results by coming ten times over the course of a year. That's not nearly enough consistency to make a difference!

So that pricing wasn't serving my client because it was basically a waste of her money at that point. It wasn't serving me because I was just getting frustrated having to repeat the same material with her every time she came in and not seeing any progress. It wasn't serving my family because it made my income really unreliable. It wasn't actually serving anyone.

But I didn't believe that I could ask my client to pay more and commit to a training schedule, so that's what I did for a long time.

When I started to change how I looked at this, I had to go back to service. I know, from years of experience, that people need to come a minimum of one time/week for movement training if it's going to make a difference in their lives. Less often than that, and we're just starting over every time. I've tried it many times, and I've never seen it work.

I knew that in order for my clients to get better results (and for me to be a happier teacher and for my income to reliably support my family), they needed to be coming weekly. So I stopped charging for ten-packs and started charging a monthly fee for weekly lessons. And by the way, I raised my rates by fifty percent when I made that change.

Did I lose some clients? Yes, I did. For some clients, it was the nudge that they needed to realize that it was time to move on, and some clients transitioned to other instructors at my studio who were still using the old model of packages.

When I reflected later, I realized that all of the clients who had moved on were the ones that I no longer felt clearly drawn to working with in my heart. They were all lovely people, but when pressed, we both realized that they were better served by moving on. The change of rates helped to clarify this.

And the clients who stuck with me were the ones who were really committed to making a change in their lives. They showed up consistently, ready to work. They did the homework I gave them. I became a much happier, more inspired, more energized teacher for them; they loved working with me more than ever, and they saw greater results than they ever had.

Make it Work for You

What I want you to understand from this chapter is how you can use your rates to be of greater service. I'm not saying that you need to use the exact business model that I used, but I do want you to challenge your own beliefs about money and how it can facilitate change.

I've invested in many coaching and self-development programs over the years. What I notice is that I consistently get the greatest results from the ones that I invest the most in. I often don't even complete the ones that are at a very low price point.

I've also noticed how clarifying a high price point is for me as buyer. If I'm considering investing in something at a low price point then it's easier to say, "Well, I guess I'll give it a try and if I'm not feeling it then I'll just stop." When something has a high price point, then I really ask myself, "Is this what I want to invest in and is now really the time?" It actually encourages me to make a much more empowered choice, and I show up so much more for what I've invested in as a result.

On the flip side, if someone pays me $100 for a service and someone else pays me $1,000 for a service, then I'm going to be much more invested in making sure that the person paying for the $1,000 service has a great experience. Charging more makes me a better teacher and coach by motivating me to be on top of my game.

I can't tell you exactly what business model will work for you, but what I can tell you is that you need to carefully look at what rates you need to charge in order to create a balanced situation in your business. To explore this further ask yourself:

1. What results do your clients really want to receive from you, and what will it take to get those results?
2. What investment will prompt your clients to commit to showing up for themselves?
3. What do you need to charge so that you can work in a way that is sustainable for your energy?
4. What amount would make you feel really, delightfully supported?

5. What income would allow you to be of greatest
    service to your family and loved ones?

Use the FORWARD method to explore each of these
questions, and remember to be open to whatever arises!

CHAPTER 11

THE EXCAVATION

The number one challenge that I see my clients run into when they start making the changes that they really desire in their lives and the one thing that stops them the most reliably is that it doesn't feel the way they thought it would feel.

We set out to make these changes because we want to feel a certain way—happier, calmer, more spacious, more relaxed, safer. We may not even realize that this is what's happening, but under the surface, we've decided that this is how we want to feel, and as soon as we do that our brains are going to start paying attention to whether we feel that way for evidence of whether this new direction is working.

The problem with this is that it will never feel better in the beginning. I wish I could wave a magic wand for you and magically your transition would be completely comfortable and feel natural right away, but that just isn't how it works. And when we don't feel happier, calmer, etc., then our brains will decide that this isn't working and will start telling us to quit.

This quitting voice sounds like, "Yes, I know this process has worked for lots of other people, but clearly it's not going to work for you, so you might as well just give up now before you make yourself look any more foolish than you already look."

That voice sounds so logical when it comes up, but I promise you that you can make this change. It is possible to balance your work with a healthy life.

Here's the key: Every part of your life as it currently exists, right now, is in your comfort zone. Even if you are really suffering right now, that suffering is a part of your current comfort zone because that is what you are used to. Making the changes you desire requires stepping out of your comfort zone. So even if you are stepping toward something you really want, you're going to feel super uncomfortable as you start moving toward it.

This is natural, but it feels really counterintuitive while you are going through it, and frequently, this is where I see people stop.

You will find other excuses like, "I don't have enough time" or "I don't know what to do" or "I'm confused" or "I'm overwhelmed" or "I'm too scared" or "I don't have enough money." And everyone in your life will believe those excuses. They will be perfectly acceptable reasons to stay where you are. But if you truly know in your heart that you can't keep going the way you are, then you cannot afford to believe those excuses.

This is where you are probably going to need to recruit help. I've really never seen anyone get through this stage without the support of an experienced guide like a coach or counsellor. This is because you are trying to navigate all of your blind spots and old patterns while, at the same time, it feels like you are dying.

And that's true; you are dying! The person who you used to be has to die to make way for the rebirth of the new person that you are becoming.

This is an ongoing process—it won't be done all in one go—but your goal is that each time you come back to the same place, you have a new perspective, you recognize it faster, and you move past it faster. If you work in this way, then your path becomes a spiral, going upward. If you don't learn to recognize your patterns and excuses for what they are, then you'll get caught in a circle and just go around and around forever.

The old habits will be so sneaky about how they try to come back. I'll give you an example from my own life.

Just this last week, there was an evening when I had planned to work on this book. On this particular evening, I was really tired. I'd had a full day of teaching, coaching, and meetings, and on top of that, I was recovering from jet lag. I was really too tired to write, but I felt like I should still do it.

One of the big patterns I've needed to reprogram through doing this process for myself is a pattern of overwork. Work addiction is something that I learned very young, and it worked well in a lot of ways until I got to the point where I was literally having a nervous breakdown as a result of my overwork.

I've been creating a new and healthy pattern around work for myself for years now and rarely fall into the overwork trap any more, but on this particular evening, I found myself really intensely reading Facebook. Understand, I wasn't just scanning posts; my body was forward, my eyes were super focused, I could feel all of my energy going into the screen— everything about me said, "I'm serious about this thing that I'm doing!"

The moment I noticed it, I just burst out laughing! Here was my work addiction trying to make another appearance. If I was honest with myself, I was too tired to work on the book that evening, but I hadn't been able to give myself permission to let go of that particular task. And so instead, some crafty part of me had created a job that I had enough energy to do (intensely reading Facebook) so I could still feel like I was working.

Now, I've been doing this work for years, so as soon as I recognized what I was going on, it was easy to drop that and go spend a little quality time with my husband before bed instead. But in the past, that wasn't so easy. If I stopped doing work (or "work" like I'd been doing that evening), then I would feel super uneasy or I'd experience a lot of guilt. My mind would go blank, and I had no idea what to do instead of the work. Not working actually felt a lot more uncomfortable than working.

You may think this story sounds silly, but if you are finding yourself overworked or feeling out of control in your own business, then you probably have some of these underlying patterns or addictions going on as well.

When you make a change, it's less about doing something new and more about changing the fundamental pattern that got you here in the first place.

I had to actually confront my work addiction and understand all of the reasons why I had chosen it and why it had been a good idea before I was able to really have a new experience.

This work is like excavation, and if you haven't been able to make a lasting shift in your life yet, then this is probably the key piece that is holding you back.

Doing the excavation work is not comfortable, but I promise you that it is worth it. As a result of doing this work, I find that I enjoy my relationships so much more and feel so much more present for them. I find delight in my life where I wouldn't have noticed it in the past. And I also show up in such a more rested and giving place for my clients. It has made me a much better healer.

There will always be reasons not to do this work—you may feel like you don't have enough time, you may be worried about whether you'll have enough money, you may not believe it will work for you, or you may feel like it's too selfish. All of these are just forms of resistance to keep you stuck where you are now.

If you are finding that it's harder to make this shift than you had realized, I just want you to know that there is nothing wrong with you. Keep going! Get help if you need it. There is gold on the other side.

Y ou've come a long way since you started this book! Let's take a look back at what you've learned. I've created a quick reference guide for you to help you quickly review your tools.

First Aid for Healers

Any time you find yourself overwhelmed, exhausted, heading into burnout, or needing a break, you can go to your version of The Cabin. This is a great place to rest, refresh, and renew yourself. The more you get to know your own energy, the earlier you'll recognize the warning signs, so you can take this time for yourself before you are in critical condition.

Be Your Own Hero

Notice when you are waiting for someone else to fix a situation for you. This is a red flag that you've shifted out of empowered thinking and into martyr or victim mentality. With compassion, notice what responsibility you are avoiding. What are you afraid of? How do you benefit by staying stuck in this situation? Then make an empowered choice about how you want to respond to the situation.

Your Practice

Use your daily practice for self-correction, for tuning into your intention and inspiration, and to renew your own energy. Know your reason for why you do your practice so that you can stay strong in it even when you want to quit.

Working with Resistance, Not Through It

The more you try to push through resistance, the stronger it gets. When you notice resistance practice CLARA, center yourself, listen, affirm what you hear, respond, and then add information. If you don't feel the resistance start to shift or transform, then go back to listening some more or get another perspective.

Moving FORWARD

Making new choices requires a new perspective. Use the FORWARD method to help you see new possibilities: Focus on your intention; open your awareness; relax your body; what do you notice; allow it to be OK; receive guidance; decide and trust. At first, you will need to set aside time to practice this method, but as you get more skillful, you'll be able to use it for a check-in at any time during your day.

Working with Your Energy

Having a new experience requires taking new actions. Pay attention to your energy and make choices that are aligned with it; then put those choices into action! In order to bring your business into balance, you'll want to pay special attention to how you are using your time to build a schedule that is in alignment with your energy.

Using Money to Serve

Rethink your fees based on how they can be of the highest service to your purpose, to your clients, and to your loved ones. Give yourself permission to release old beliefs about money, and price your services in a way that is aligned with creating a sustainable life for yourself and offering your greatest service to your clients.

Excavation

You didn't end up in your current situation by accident. Some part of you chose this pattern for reasons that made good sense at the time. Do the excavation work to understand why you created this pattern so you can consciously create a new pattern and so you won't end up in this same situation again. Get support to help you see your blind spots and walk with you through the challenges.

The View

I believe that the truest measure of success in our healing businesses is our own ability to live full and healthy lives. You can really only heal yourself, but through doing your own healing work, you will offer healing to everyone around you.

The reason why I'm so passionate about helping healers get their own work in balance is because we have power beyond what I think most of us realize. I look around the world and I see a lot of people suffering. I see pain; I see divisions—and you know what that world needs? It needs healers! It needs people who are ready to step up and serve others to transform suffering into meaning and to heal old wounds.

But I truly believe that we can't do the work we are meant to do when we ourselves are depleted or working from a martyr mindset. By stepping into our own true power, we become the beacons of the possibility that our work truly offers. Empowered choice is contagious. It offers a kind of freedom that many people don't realize is available to them at every moment of their lives.

My dream is to live in a world of people who are ready to make empowered choices and work together to build a world where we can all flourish. It's a lofty dream, I know, but by showing up as the models of what is possible, the healers of this world can help to make that vision real. Imagine the ripple effect we could have if every healer showed up to their work fully inspired and as the best version of themselves. This is what inspires me in this work. I would love to have you join me in it!

ACKNOWLEDGMENTS

All of my thanks and gratitude...

...to all of my wonderful clients, both in movement and in coaching—thank you for sharing your lives, your struggles, and your victories with me. You are my inspiration to always bring my best self to my work.

...to my colleagues at Joy. I wish for each of you to grow and thrive in your own work and journeys!

...to Sura Kim, Michael Patrick, Nic Askew, Heather Clark, and Lisa Lansing for your mentorship.

...to Jay Sandweiss for sharing your journey with me with humor and compassion and for inspiring my own journey.

...to Michelle Segar for your enthusiastic yes followed immediately by heartfelt guidance and support.

…to my book launch team for your support and especially to Jill Brown for sharing word of this book far and wide and Liza Baker for her eagle-eyed and thorough feedback.

…to the Morgan James Publishing team: Special thanks to David Hancock, CEO & Founder for believing in me and my message. To my Author Relations Manager, Margo Toulouse, thanks for making the process seamless and easy. Many more thanks to everyone else, but especially Jim Howard, Bethany Marshall, and Nickcole Watkins.

…to Angela Lauria, Tami Stackelhouse, the rest of the team, and my cohort at The Author Incubator for holding space for me through this journey. I'm so honored to be a part of this group of superhumans!

…to Moriah Howell for being the best cheerleader and editor a first-time author could wish for.

…to Petey, Laramie, Rue, and Dexter for being my daily teachers of unconditional love.

…to my parents for your generous support and for always encouraging me to live the life that truly calls my heart.

…and to my husband for being my best friend and ally.

ABOUT THE AUTHOR

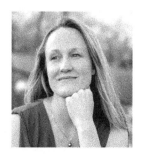 Heather Glidden is a certified integrative coach and the owner of multiple successful healing arts studios.

Her mission is to free healers in their businesses so they can make the difference they are truly in this world to make. She serves her clients in all aspects of building a thriving business in a way that feels good to them.

Heather's approach combines life coaching with deep listening, meditation, energy healing, practical business knowledge, and research-based tools to break through limiting beliefs.

Using this approach with her clients has allowed them to experience more joy and to up-level their businesses with ease.

Heather lives in Ann Arbor, Michigan. When she isn't working, you might find her dancing, walking her two dogs, playing board games with friends, or going on adventures with her husband.

Website: www.heatherglidden.com

THANK YOU!

Thank you for reading *Thrive in Your Healing Business*! This isn't the end but rather the beginning of a new way of life for you. I sincerely hope this book has provided you with the tools, inspiration, and encouragement you need to bring your healing business into balance.

It's one thing to read about balancing your business and quite another to actually do the work to make it happen. I've created a free training to help you get started. You can download it at my website here: www.heatherglidden.com/thrive

I'm wishing you everything wonderful as you undertake this new journey. You've got this! You know where to find me if you need support.

CPSIA information can be obtained
at www.ICGtesting.com
Printed in the USA
LVHW041151271219
641843LV00001B/118/P

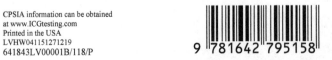